SAINT-FRANCES
GUIDE TO
PSYCHIATRY

SAINT-FRANCES GUIDE TO PSYCHIATRY

Malia McCarthy, M.D.

Child and Adolescent Psychiatry Fellow
Yale Child Study Center
Yale University School of Medicine
New Haven, Connecticut

Mary B. O'Malley, M.D., Ph.D.

Assistant Attending Physician, Department of Psychiatry
Sleep Medicine Consultant
Norwalk Hospital, Norwalk Connecticut
Clinical Instructor in the Department of Psychiatry
New York University
New York, New York

Series Editor:

Sanjay Saint, M.D., M.P.H.

Assistant Professor of Medicine
Division of General Medicine
University of Michigan Medical School
Ann Arbor, Michigan

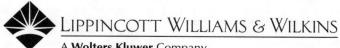

LIPPINCOTT WILLIAMS & WILKINS
A **Wolters Kluwer** Company
Philadelphia • Baltimore • New York • London
Buenos Aires • Hong Kong • Sydney • Tokyo

Editor: Elizabeth A. Nieginski
Editorial Director: Julie P. Scardiglia
Development Editor: Emilie Linkins
Associate Development Editor: Elizabeth Lowe
Managing Editor: Darrin Kiessling
Marketing Manager: Kelley Ray

Printed in the United States of America

Library of Congress Cataloging-in-Publication Data

McCarthy, Malia.
  Saint-Frances guide to psychiatry / Malia McCarthy, Mary B. O'Malley, Sanjay Saint.
    p. ; cm.
  Includes index.
  ISBN 0-683-30661-8
  1. Psychiatry—Handbooks, manuals, etc. 2. Psychiatry—Oulines, syllabi, etc.
I. Title: Guide to psychiatry. II. O'Malley, Mary B. III. Saint, Sanjay. IV. Title.
  [DNLM: 1. Mental Disorders—Handbooks. 2. Mental Disorders—Outlines.
WM 18.2 M4786s 2000]
  RC454 .M324 2000
  616.89—dc21

00-045340

We'd like to hear from you! If you have comments or suggestions regarding this Lippincott Williams & Wilkins title, please contact us at the appropriate customer service number listed below, or send correspondence to **book_comments@lww.com**. If possible, please remember to include your mailing address, phone number, and a reference to the book title and author in your message. To purchase additional copies of this book call our customer service department at **(800) 638-3030** or fax orders to **(301) 824-7390**. International customers should call **(301) 714-2324**.

01 02 03
1 2 3 4 5 6 7 8 9 10

Dedication

To Emma, for whom I wish a lifetime of joy
in learning, and to Brandon,
whose love makes all things possible.
Malia McCarthy

To Ed, whose love and support always
helps me find focus, and to Miriah, Becca,
Dylan, and Liam, with love.
Mary B. O'Malley

To my family and friends.
Sanjay Saint

SAINT-FRANCES GUIDE TO PSYCHIATRY

Contents

✦

PART IV. SUBSTANCE ABUSE

PART V. MOOD DISORDERS

PART VI. ANXIETY DISORDERS

PART VII. DISSOCIATIVE DISORDERS

PART VIII. PERSONALITY DISORDERS

PART IX. CONSULTATION–LIAISON ISSUES

Contributors

Hugh Bases, M.D.
Developmental/Behavioral Pediatrics Fellow
Yale University School of Medicine
New Haven, Connecticut
Chapter 44, Elimination Disorders

Leslie Bogen, J.D., Ph.D.
Instructor of Psychology in Psychiatry
Weill Medical College
Cornell University
New York, New York
Clinical Instructor
Yale Child Study Center
Yale University School of Medicine
New Haven, Connecticut
Chapter 4, Psychiatric Treatment

Sharon Eberstein, M.D.
Assistant Clinical Professor of Psychiatry
Columbia University College of Physicians and Surgeons
Attending Psychiatrist
St. Luke's–Roosevelt Hospital Center
New York, New York
Chapter 9, Overview of Psychosis
Chapter 10, Schizophrenia
Chapter 11, Antipsychotic Medications

Rajiv Gulati, M.D.
Clinical Instructor in Psychiatry
New York University School of Medicine
New York, New York
Chapter 35, Human Sexuality and Sexual Dysfunction
Chapter 36, Paraphilias
Chapter 37, Gender Identity Disorder

Marianne T. Guschwan, M.D.
Clinical Assistant Professor of Psychiatry
New York University School of Medicine
Unit Chief, Detoxification Unit
Bellevue Hospital
New York, New York
Chapter 12, Alcohol Abuse and Dependence
Chapter 13, Opioid Abuse and Dependence
Chapter 14, Other Drugs of Abuse

Silvia Hafliger, M.D.
Assistant Clinical Professor of Psychiatry
Columbia University College of Physicians and Surgeons
Attending Consultation Liaison Psychiatrist
Columbia-Presbyterian Medical Center
New York, New York
Chapter 24, Capacity Assessment
Chapter 25, Delirium
Chapter 26, Death & Grief
Chapter 27, Unexplained Somatic Symptoms and Somatoform Disorders

John Holmberg, Psy.D.
Child and Adolescent Psychology Fellow
Yale Child Study Center
Yale University School of Medicine
New Haven, Connecticut
Chapter 38, Development

Lori Plutchik, M.D.
Clinical Instructor of Psychiatry
Albert Einstein College of Medicine
Department of Consultation Liaison Psychiatry and Behavioral
    Medicine
Beth Israel Medical Center
New York, New York
Chapter 28, Psychiatric Aspects of HIV Disease

Laura Ross, M.D.
Clinical Instructor of Psychiatry
New York University School of Medicine
New York, New York
*Chapter 29, Psychiatric Disorders During Pregnancy and
    Postpartum*

Preface

The Saint-Frances Guide to Psychiatry addresses psychiatry using much the same format as the other books in the *Saint-Frances Guide* series. It distills the most clinically useful information in inpatient and outpatient psychiatry. It can function as a rotation "survival guide," as a text to use in preparing for exams, and as an easily-accessed reference for practitioners in other fields of medicine. *The Saint-Frances Guide to Psychiatry* will be useful to medical students and psychiatry residents early in their training, as well as to clinical psychologists and clinical psychology trainees, psychiatric social workers, and psychiatric nurses.

This pocket-sized book consists of short, easily-mastered chapters and includes memory aids such as mnemonics, "hot keys," and simple charts. A busy medical student or trainee (and there is no other type) will find this book useful in keeping up with patient care. When informed that she will be treating a newly admitted patient with a dissociative disorder, for example, the clinician can quickly locate the relevant chapter in the book, review the five-minute synopsis on the subject (which includes clinical manifestations, differential diagnosis, approach to the patient, treatment, and follow-up), and commit the diagnostic criteria to memory via a brief mnemonic. The contents of each chapter focus upon the most clinically useful information. "Hot keys" call the clinician's attention to key issues. Each chapter concludes with a few key references, as new practitioners often do not have the time or experience to discern the most relevant and concise literature from the thousands of listings on computer databases.

The Saint-Frances Guide to Psychiatry is organized to include the most fundamental issues at the outset, and then proceeds to cover the topics that students are frequently expected to master. The introductory section includes chapters on the mental status exam and psychiatric treatment in general. Next, disorders often treated in inpatient and then outpatient settings are covered, such as psychoses, mood disorders, and anxiety disorders. Specialized topics in psychiatry are covered later, such as consultation-liaison issues, sleep disorders, child and adolescent psychiatry, and issues in geriatric psychiatry. Within this framework, brief chapters on related topics are grouped. For example, the chapter on psychosis and its differential diagnosis is grouped with chapters on antipsychotic medications and schizophrenia.

The Saint-Frances Guide to Psychiatry is unique among clinical manuals in psychiatry in that every chapter was reviewed for clarity, simplicity, and comprehensibility by a non-psychiatrist physician. Dr. Saint, a general internist and co-author of the very successful *Saint-Frances Guide to Inpatient Medicine* and *Saint-Frances Guide to Outpatient Medicine,* served the important role of assuring that everything in this book could be easily understood by the non-psychiatrist. Because *The Saint-Frances Guide to Psychiatry* stems from such a collaboration, we believe it is a uniquely user-friendly, practical guide to psychiatry. We hope this book will add to your confidence and enjoyment in treating psychiatric patients, and to your understanding of and interest in this exciting field!

Acknowledgments

I would like to acknowledge the teaching and support of Dorothy Stubbe, M.D., Joe Woolston, M.D., Fred Volkmar, M.D., Sandra Boltax-Stern, M.D., and Samuel Ritvo, M.D., as well as the many other fine teachers and clinicians at the Yale Child Study Center Child and Adolescent Psychiatry Training Program and the New York University General Psychiatry Residency Training Program.

—Malia McCarthy

I would like to thank Joyce Walsleben, Ph.D., R.N., and David Rapoport, M.D. of the New York University Sleep Disorders Center for their exceptional teaching and support. I am also grateful to my colleagues and mentors at New York University's General Psychiatry Training Program for their contributions to this book, and to my education.

—Mary B. O'Malley

I would like to acknowledge the overall support and patience of my wife, Veronica Saint, in helping me complete this book. I would also like to acknowledge the secretarial support provided by Carolyn Campbell in the Division of General Medicine at the University of Michigan Medical School.

—Sanjay Saint

Finally, we would all like to acknowledge Emilie Linkins, Development Editor at Lippincott Williams & Wilkins, for her superb editorial work and for keeping us on track, Elizabeth Nieginski, Senior Acquisitions Editor at Lippincott Williams & Wilkins, for continuing her outstanding work in shepherding the Saint-Frances series, and Managing Editor Darrin Kiessling.

PART I

INTRODUCTION

1. DSM-IV™

I DSM-IV is the fourth edition of the *Diagnostic and Statistical Manual of Mental Disorders,* copyright 1994 by the American Psychiatric Association (APA). The DSM-IV **lists diagnostic criteria for each psychiatric disorder.**

A. Making diagnoses according to DSM-IV criteria is important for purposes of **research and communication** among mental health professionals.
   1. The DSM-IV criteria **provide a common vocabulary.** For example, separate groups researching schizophrenia can compare findings, knowing that the same diagnostic criteria were used in patient selection.
   2. Or, when a clinician discharges a patient with a diagnosis of "schizophrenia," this **communicates to subsequent caregivers** how a patient's difficulties were conceptualized and gives some notion of the patient's clinical features at that point in time.
   3. In addition, DSM-IV diagnoses are important for **billing purposes.**
B. DSM diagnoses represent an **evolving body of knowledge.** Diagnostic criteria are determined by the Task Force on DSM-IV and other committees and work groups of the APA and reflect the published literature. The previous edition was the revised third edition, or DSM-III-R, published in 1987. The first edition was the DSM-I, published in 1952.
C. **DSM diagnoses are descriptive.** The DSM criteria for diagnoses focus on clinical manifestations and are largely unconcerned with the etiology of the various disorders.

II **"Mental disorder"** refers to any behavioral or psychological syndrome that causes clinically significant distress or disability or that places the individual at risk of death, pain, disability, or serious loss of freedom.

A. The diagnosis of a mental disorder has important clinical and prognostic implications.

B. Many patients have more than one diagnosis.

C. It is important to assemble a list of differential diagnoses upon initial evaluation of a patient and then to carefully consider each possibility.

HOT KEY A psychiatric diagnosis is only one way to conceptualize a patient. Beyond diagnosis, there is an enormous amount of information that is unique to the individual patient. Such information is important in understanding the patient psychologically and instituting appropriate treatment.

III **MULTIAXIAL ASSESSMENT** is used in the DSM-IV. This involves categorizing information about a patient along five axes, which are listed below. In addition to the psychiatric diagnoses, the multiaxial assessment includes information about the patient's medical conditions, stressors, and overall level of functioning. This system reflects a biopsychosocial approach.

Axis I: Clinical Disorders and Other Conditions That May Be a Focus of Clinical Attention

Axis II: Personality Disorders and Mental Retardation

Axis III: General Medical Conditions (which are relevant to understanding of the psychiatric condition)

Axis IV: Psychosocial and Environmental Problems

Axis V: Global Assessment of Functioning (GAF) Scale (varies from a low of 0 to a high of 100, which would apply to a patient who has superior functioning in a wide range of activities). This can be useful for following progress with treatment.

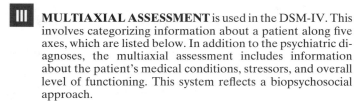

TABLE 1-1. Example of How to Record a DSM-IV Multiaxial Evaluation		
Axis I	296.23	Major Depressive Disorder, Single Episode, Severe Without Psychotic Features
	305.00	Alcohol Abuse
Axis II	301.6	Dependent Personality Disorder
Axis III		None
Axis IV		Unemployment
Axis V		GAF=45 (on admission)
		GAF=65 (at discharge)

GAF = Global Assessment of Functioning Scale.

Table 1-1 gives an example of how to record a DSM-IV multiaxial evaluation. The appendix at the back of this book gives a complete listing of the DSM-IV classification.

References

American Psychiatric Association: *Diagnostic and Statistical Manual of Mental Disorders,* 4th ed. Washington, DC, American Psychiatric Association, 1994.

Jensen PS, Hoagwood K: The book of names: DSM-IV in context. *Dev Psychopathol* 9(2):231–249, 1997.

Regier DA, Kaelber CT, Rae DS, et al: Limitations of diagnostic criteria and assessment instruments for mental disorders. Implications for research and policy. *Arch Gen Psychiatry* 55(2):109–115, 1998.

Spitzer RL, Wakefield JC: DSM-IV diagnostic criterion for clinical significance: Does it help solve the false positives problem? *Am J Psychiatry* 156(12):1856–1864, 1999.

2. The Psychiatric Interview and Presentation

I **INTRODUCTION.** The diagnostic psychiatric interview serves two major purposes: collection of historical data and performance of the mental status examination. While taking the history, the physician is actively assessing the various components of the patient's mental status (see Chapter 3). Although these two functions are performed concurrently, they are discussed here separately for clarity.

II **PRESENTATION OF THE PSYCHIATRIC PATIENT.** The psychiatric patient is presented in the following order, which is similar to the presentation of the medical or surgical patient. The information may or may not be collected from the patient in this order:

A. Identifying information

Mr. R. is a 30-year-old Hispanic male mechanic who lives in a rented apartment with his mother and stepfather. The patient served as the sole source of historical information.

B. Chief complaint

The patient was self-referred to the clinic 2 weeks ago complaining that "My heart keeps racing and I can't breathe, and I'm afraid I'm going to die."

HOT
KEY

It is always best to try to use the patient's own words for the chief complaint.

C. History of present illness (HPI). This is the main part of the interview.

1. **The nature, duration, and severity of symptoms** should be quantified as much as possible.
2. **Stressors should be identified** that may be related to onset of symptoms or relapse.
3. **The meaning of the symptoms to the patient** should be understood. For example, one patient may attribute medical meaning to panic symptoms, and another patient may fear that her panic symptoms mean she is "going crazy."
4. The **HPI includes all pertinent positives and negatives.** For example, if a patient is presenting with panic symptoms, all DSM-IV criteria for panic disorder should be explored. Symptoms of other disorders in the differential should be asked about, and related disorders should be screened for.

PATIENT PROFILE

HPI: The patient, Mr. R., was in his usual state of health until the anniversary of his father's death 3 weeks ago, when he began to experience 20-minute episodes of intense fearfulness, sweating, tightness in his chest, and palpitations, which prevented him from engaging in other activities. He saw his internist who did an EKG and blood work and told him he was "perfectly healthy." The patient expresses a great deal of confusion about his symptoms as well as fear that he may have a heart attack, as his father did. He experienced no trembling, nausea, dizziness, paresthesias, dissociative symptoms, hot or cold flashes, or fear of going crazy. He has no symptoms of agoraphobia. He denied obsessive thoughts, compulsive rituals, depressed mood, or loss of energy.

D. **Past psychiatric history.** This should describe:
   1. **Age at onset of illness and presentation** at that time
   2. Any **previous inpatient and outpatient treatment** including duration, nature of treatment, effectiveness, compliance, and relapse factors
   3. **Drug, alcohol, and tobacco use** including symptoms of abuse or dependence and any associated treatment
   4. Any **history of suicidal behavior** (see Chapter 7) or **assaultiveness**
E. **Past medical history.** This should include:
   1. Major illnesses and hospitalizations
   2. Current medications and allergies
   3. Any history of head injuries with loss of consciousness or any history of seizure disorders
   4. Human immunodeficiency virus (HIV) testing and risk factors for HIV infection

     5. History of tuberculosis

     6. Last menstrual period (for female patients)

F. Family history. This should include any information about blood relatives (i.e., parents, siblings, children, aunts, uncles, cousins, or grandparents) with any history of known psychiatric illness, psychiatric hospitalizations, psychiatric treatment, suicide attempts, drug or alcohol abuse, major medical illnesses, or "trouble with the law."

G. Social and developmental history. The following factors are relevant to the evaluation:

     1. Education—how much schooling the patient has completed; whether the patient attended "special ed" or "regular" classes

     2. Upbringing—who raised the patient; description of parents and any siblings; history of any physical, sexual, or verbal abuse (e.g., "Were you ever hurt by an adult—either touched inappropriately or hit so that marks were left on your body?")

     3. Adult life—age at which the patient left home; history of any adult romantic relationships or marriage; marital status; sexual orientation (e.g., "When you have sex, is it usually with men or women or both?"); any children and if so, who has custody, and whether any of the children have been in any "trouble with the law"

     4. Work and military history and **current source of income**

     5. Religion, ethnicity, and **language** spoken at home

     6. Supportive people currently in the patient's life

     7. Activities the patient enjoys currently

H. Mental status examination (see Chapter 3)

I. Differential diagnosis: a list of possible diagnoses based on currently available information

J. Formulation: one or two sentences reflecting a biopsychosocial formulation—the biologic, psychological, and social factors that help explain the patient's current presentation.

FORMULATION: "Mr. R. is a 30-year-old man with a history of social deprivation and exposure to multiple traumas, strongly genetically loaded for anxiety disorders, who presents with acute panic symptoms apparently precipitated by the recent anniversary of his father's death. The symptoms are highly distressing to Mr. R., who fears that they may mean that he, too, is having a heart attack."

K. Work-up and treatment plan or **disposition plan** (see Chapter 4 and Chapter 8 IV) may include additional diagnostic interviews, family assessment, physical or neurologic examination, or psychological, neurologic, or laboratory tests as indicated. The plan often includes **checking collateral history sources,** including family, friends, current health care providers, and old records, as soon as possible. This is particularly important if you are concerned about whether the patient might be dangerous or about his ability to care for himself and follow treatment recommendations, or about possible substance abuse or malingering, or if treatment decisions need to be made imminently. Always document that you have checked, or attempted to check, collateral history sources.

III IMPORTANT ASPECTS OF THE PSYCHIATRIC INTERVIEW

A. The initial consultation generally lasts 30 minutes to 1 hour, depending on the circumstances. It is important to explain the purpose and anticipated length of the interview to the patient at the outset. Often, collecting the historical data in roughly the same order in which it is presented in section II helps to organize the interview. For example, the clinician could approach the interview as follows: "Before we talk about why you've come today, I'd like to ask you a few questions. Please tell me your name. How old are you? Where do you live? How do you support yourself?"

B. After collecting identifying information, the interview usually proceeds with **open-ended questions,** for example, "How can we help you in the clinic today?" This is a good opportunity to assess elements of the mental status such as speech, relatedness, and thought form (see Chapter 3) as well as to discern which of the symptoms or why the evaluation is important to the patient. After the patient has had several minutes to respond, you should have some idea about whether the patient will be able to provide a coherent history. In general, the more disorganized the patient, the more the interviewer will need to give structure to the interview by asking pointed questions.

> **HOT KEY**
> Diagnostic interviews generally proceed from more open-ended questions (e.g., "Tell me about yourself.") to more closed-ended questions (e.g., "What is today's date?").

Often, closed-ended questions are also used to follow up information given in response to open-ended questions.

C. Usually, the interview concludes by giving the patient a chance to ask questions. The interviewer then provides **feedback** and a

brief discussion of the plan, conveying a sense of confidence and, if possible, hope (e.g., "You've been very helpful talking to me about so many difficult subjects. It sounds like you've been having a really difficult time lately. The type of problem you're having often responds well to treatment. You've made a very good decision in seeking help. Right now, I'm going to discuss what you told me with the rest of the team. I'll come back in 20 minutes, and then we'll talk about how this clinic can best help you.").

D. To conduct an effective interview, **good rapport with the patient** is essential. Good rapport can be established with an approach of courtesy, respect, and adoption of a nonjudgmental and helpful attitude. This may be more difficult than it sounds, but there are general guidelines for doing so, which are easy to remember. A psychiatrist who "CARED" is usually able to develop good rapport with patients.

Guidelines for Establishing Rapport with Patients ("CARED")

Communication—both verbal and nonverbal—is very important, and the interviewer should be attuned to this

Attend to that which is important to the patient

Respect the patient and his life experiences; imagine and try to understand what it is like to live your patient's life for 24 hours

Expected answers should not be suggested by the physician because patients usually want to please the physician and thus may provide the answer that they feel is expected of them

Dignity—psychiatric patients are often looked down upon in society; try not to inadvertently convey this attitude in your interview. Wear professional attire, and seat the patient in a chair of equal height. Address the patient by "Mr." or "Ms."

References

American Psychiatric Association: Practice guidelines for psychiatric evaluation of adults. *Am J Psychiatry* 152:63a–80a, 1995.

Carlat DJ: The psychiatric review of symptoms: A screening tool for family physicians. *Am Fam Physician* 58(7):1617–1624, 1998.

Coupey SM: Interviewing adolescents. *Pediatr Clin North Am* 44(6):1349–1364, 1997.

*Engel GL: The clinical application of the biopsychosocial model. *Am J Psychiatry* 137:535–544, 1980.

*Perry S, Cooper AM, Michels R: The psychodynamic formulation: Its purpose, structure, and clinical application. *Am J Psychiatry* 144:543–550, 1987.

*classic reference

3. The Mental Status Examination

I **INTRODUCTION.** The **mental status examination (MSE)** is the psychiatrist's equivalent of the physical examination.

A. It is an **objective assessment of the patient's mental functioning.**

> **HOT** ▶ **KEY**
>
> The MSE reflects the patient's mental status **at the particular point in time at which it is performed.** This differs from the history, which includes historical information about mental functioning.

B. In assessing mental status, it is important for the psychiatrist to **observe both verbal and nonverbal communication.**

C. The MSE is **performed concurrently with the psychiatric interview** (see Chapter 2), but it is presented separately.

> **HOT** ▶ **KEY**
>
> The patient's own words and specific behaviors should be recorded when taking the MSE.

II **THE MENTAL STATUS EXAMINATION**

A. **Appearance.** A physical description of the patient should be recorded so that he could be picked out of a room full of people. The description should include physical characteristics, apparent age, grooming, and eye contact.

B. **Attitude** toward interviewer. A description of the patient's attitude might be, for example, "cooperative," "suspicious," "eager to please," "flirtatious," or "hostile."

C. **Psychomotor status.** This refers to a patient's nonverbal behavior. Psychomotor activity may be **increased (psychomotor agitation)** or **decreased (psychomotor retardation).** The extremes of these states are **catatonic excitement** (agitated, purposeless motor activity) and **catatonic posturing** (voluntary assumption of a bizarre posture for an extended period of time). **Hyperactivity** refers to restless, often purposeless movements of the larger skeletal muscles, such as running in circles around the examination room. **Mannerisms** are repetitive, purposeless, involuntary movements, such as grimacing.

D. **Speech** refers to the **mechanical, productive components of language:**

1. **Articulation** (e.g., slurred, dysarthric)
2. **Volume** (e.g., loud, soft)
3. **Rate** (e.g., slow, rapid). A concept related to rate is that of **pressured speech.** Pressured speech is difficult to interrupt, as though a patient is responding to an internal drive to continue speaking. Pressured speech is usually rapid.
4. **Rhythm** (e.g., stammer)

E. Thought and perception

1. **Thought** has both form and content.

(a) **Thought form** in a person without psychiatric disturbance is typically **linear** or **goal directed.** Other kinds of thought form follow:

(1) **Circumstantiality**—the patient thinks circuitously but ultimately gets to the point

(2) **Tangentiality**—the patient gets side-tracked and never gets to the point

(3) **Derailment**—speech may initially appear linear but with repeated shift in focus

(4) **Loosening of associations**—the connections between thoughts are not apparent to the listener

(5) **Word salad or incoherence**—no apparent connection between thoughts, even within a sentence

(6) **Flight of ideas**—thoughts are connected but occur so rapidly that it is difficult for the listener to keep up and understand

(7) **Thought blocking**—a sudden interruption of speech with a subsequent inability to continue

(8) **Neologism**—the patient makes up his own words, for example, "wonderphenom"

(9) **Clang association**—associations are via rhyme

(10) **Vague**—thoughts are not well elaborated

(b) **Thought content** assessment includes evaluation for:

(1) **Suicidal** or **homicidal ideation** (see Chapter 7 II B and Chapter 8 II C)

(2) **Delusions,** which are **fixed false beliefs** and may be of many types, including **paranoid, grandiose, somatic, erotomanic,** and **bizarre.** Other types of delusions include **thought broadcasting** (belief that others can hear one's thoughts) and **thought insertion** (belief that others are placing thoughts in one's mind).

(3) **Paranoid ideation** and **grandiosity** refer to such content not of delusional proportions

(4) **Ideas of reference** involve the feeling that others

(e.g., on radio or television) are talking to or about the patient
- **(5) Preoccupations** (e.g., somatic)
- **(6) Obsessions and compulsions**
- **(7) Phobias** (e.g., social phobia, agoraphobia, claustrophobia)
- **(8) Poverty of content**

2. **Perceptual disturbances** include hallucinations, which are usually either **auditory** or **visual,** but may also be **tactile** or **olfactory.** Patients are often reluctant to disclose hallucinations, but **"internal preoccupation"** or **"responding to internal stimuli"** (talking to oneself) may suggest their presence. **Derealization** is the feeling that one's environment is unreal; **depersonalization** is the feeling that one's self is unreal.

F. Mood and affect
1. **Mood** refers to the predominant emotion that a patient experiences and is largely ascertained from the patient's subjective report. A description of the patient's mood may be "happy," "sad," "worried," or "angry."
2. **Affect** is an **objective description** of the patient's expression of emotion. Affect has many dimensions, including constricted or full **range** (e.g., the affect can be constricted to "sad," or it can be "predominantly sad but of a wider range," such as in a patient who is sad but smiling at times), **stability** (e.g., "labile" or "monotonous"), **intensity** (e.g., "flat," "blunted," or "intense"), and **appropriateness to content.**

HOT

KEY

Affect will usually vary over the course of the interview with each new idea or thought. Mood is generally more enduring.

G. Cognition. Another component of the MSE involves assessment of cognitive functioning. This usually includes the following elements:
1. **Sensorium**
   a. **Alertness** or **level of consciousness.** A description of the patient's level of consciousness could be, for example, "lethargic," "sleepy," or "alert." The level of consciousness should be noted at the outset, because it will affect the way in which the MSE will be interpreted. For example, a patient who is somnolent at the time of assessment will likely present differently when alert.
   b. **Assessing the four spheres of orientation—person, place, time,** and **situation**
2. **Attention** is the ability to focus on a task, for example, repeat-

ing a series of digits forward and backward. **Concentration** is the ability to maintain focus on an internal thought process, such as subtracting 7 from 100, then subtracting 7 from the remainder, and continuing the series to 65 ("serial sevens"). If the patient has difficulty with calculation, she might instead be asked to spell "world" forward and then backward.

3. **Memory**
   a. **Immediate memory** refers to the patient's ability to repeat the names of several items that the examiner has just recited. **Recall** is the patient's ability to repeat the items after 5 minutes.
   b. **Recent memory** refers to memory of events of past hours or days and sometimes those of past weeks.
   c. **Remote memory** refers to long-term memory and is usually evaluated by asking for historical or autobiographical information.

4. **Abstract thought** refers to the ability to shift from specific ideas to generic ones. It can be assessed by asking questions about similarities and differences and by asking for interpretations of proverbs.

5. **Intelligence** is assessed by fund of standard knowledge, vocabulary, and proverb interpretation, taking cultural and educational background into consideration.

H. **Insight** refers to the patient's awareness of her problem and its meaning.

I. **Judgment** may be assessed through hypothetical questions (e.g., "If there was a fire in a movie theater, what would you do?") or, preferably, through one's ability to set reasonable goals for one's life and approach them in an appropriate way (e.g., given his current psychiatric problems, how is the patient choosing to approach them?)

J. **Impulse control.** Is the patient able to refrain from acting on impulses over the course of the interview?

III FURTHER EXAMINATION. Depending on the patient's presentation, various parts of the MSE should be abbreviated or expanded upon. For example, in a psychotic patient, the examiner should explore more fully the various psychotic symptoms and cite both positive and negative findings. In a patient with findings suggesting delirium or dementia, one would more fully assess cognitive functioning with a "Mini-Mental State Examination" (Table 3-1).

References

Brackley MH: Mental health assessment/mental status examination. *Nurse Practitioner Forum* 8(3):105–113, 1997.

Sartorius N, Janca A: Psychiatric assessment instruments developed by the World Health Organization. *Soc Psychiatry Psychiatr Epidemiol* 31(2):55–69, 1996.

TABLE 3-1. Mini-Mental State Examination

Maximum Score	Score	

(5) __

Orientation

Ask the patient for the date. Then ask specifically for the parts omitted (e.g., "Can you also tell me what season it is?"). Award 1 point for each correct answer.

____	____	____	____	____
year	season	date	day	month

(5) __

Ask the patient in turn, "Can you tell me the name of this: floor? hospital? town? county? state?" Award 1 point for each correct answer.

____	____	____	____	____
state	county	town	hospital	floor

Registration

(3) __

Ask the patient if you may test his memory. Then say the names of 3 unrelated objects, clearly and slowly, allowing about 1 second between each. After you have named all 3 objects, ask the patient to repeat them. This first repetition determines his score (0–3), but keep repeating the objects until the patient can repeat all 3, up to 6 trials. Award 1 point for each correct answer and record the number of trials. If the patient does not eventually learn all 3 objects, recall cannot be meaningfully tested (see below).

____	____	____	____	____
				trial #

Attention and Calculation

(5) __

Ask the patient to begin with 100 and count backward by increments of 7. Stop after 5 subtractions. Award 1 point for each correct answer.

100

____	____	____	____	____
93	86	79	72	65

If the patient cannot or will not perform this task, ask him to spell "world" backward. Award 1 point for each letter named in correct order.

____	____	____	____	____
d	l	r	o	w

Recall

(3) __

Ask the patient if he can repeat 3 objects you previously asked him to remember. Award 1 point for each.

TABLE 3-1. Mini-Mental State Examination *(Continued)*

Maximum Score	Score	

Language

(2)   __   Show the patient a watch and ask him what it is. Repeat for a pencil. Award 1 point for each correct answer.

(1)   __   Ask the patient to repeat the sentence after you: "No ifs, ands or buts." Award 1 point for the correct answer.

(3)   __   Give the patient a blank sheet of paper and ask him to follow a 3 stage command: "Take this paper in your hand, fold it in half, and place it on the floor." Award 1 point for each part correctly executed.

(1)   __   Ask the patient to read the following statement and do what it says. Award 1 point if the patient performs the action correctly.

CLOSE YOUR EYES

(1)   __   Ask the patient to write a sentence for you. Do not dictate a sentence. The sentence must contain a subject and a verb, but grammar and punctuation are not necessary. Award 1 point if the patient performs the action correctly.

(1)   __   Ask the patient to copy the following design. Each figure must have 5 sides and 2 of the angles must intersect. Award 1 point if the patient performs the action correctly.

Total Score: ___

Assess the patient's level of consciousness along a continuum:

alert	drowsy	stuporous	comatose

Patient: _____   **Unit#:** _____

Examiner: _____   **Date:** _____

From Folstein MF, Folstein SE, McHugh PR: "Mini-mental state." A practical method for grading the cognitive state of patients for the clinician. *J Psychiatr Res* 12(3):189–198, 1975. Used by permission of MiniMental LLC.

4. Psychiatric Treatment

I INITIAL CONSIDERATIONS IN TREATMENT PLANNING

A. The cause of psychiatric symptoms must be identified to plan for effective treatment.

> **HOT KEY**
> Symptoms must be fully fleshed out in terms of the diagnosis, any precipitants or stressors, and the meaning of the symptoms to the individual patient. All of these factors will inform solid treatment planning.

B. Comorbidity and course

1. Psychiatric disorders may be **acute** (i.e., severe symptoms with a short course) or **chronic** (i.e., symptoms that persist for a long time).
2. The course of a psychiatric disorder may be complicated by **concomitant psychiatric disorders** (e.g., personality disorders, mental retardation).
   a. It is not unusual for certain disorders to occur together (e.g., Tourette's disorder and obsessive-compulsive disorder; depression and anxiety) because of genetic factors, similar risk factors, or because one disorder evolves into another disorder.
   b. The cause-and-effect relationship of disorders that occur together is rarely straightforward or linear. More often, a multitude of factors are involved in complicated interrelationships.
3. Patients with **medical disorders** may present with symptoms of psychiatric disorders.
4. In some cases, **psychiatric treatment** complicates the diagnostic picture. For example, agitation in a patient with schizophrenia may represent akathisia associated with antipsychotic medications or an increase in psychotic symptoms; the interventions for each would be quite different.

> **HOT KEY**
> The way in which one condition relates to others or to treatment itself should attempt to be clarified, as this underlies effective treatment planning.

II OPTIONS IN TREATMENT PLANNING

> **HOT**
>
>
>
> **KEY**
>
> In formulating a treatment plan, it is useful to organize thinking about a clinical picture by considering each component of the biopsychosocial model: the biological, psychological, and social aspects of the patient's presentation.

A. Biological interventions. Somatic treatments include pharmacological therapy, light therapy, electroconvulsive therapy (see Chapter 15 IV D), adjustment of sleep patterns, and, in extreme cases, psychosurgery.

   1. Effective pharmacological treatment requires assessing which **symptoms,** if any, may be appropriately and effectively treated with medication and recognizing the **limits of pharmacological treatment.**

   2. Most psychopharmacological medications affect neurotransmitters by targeting receptors and enzymes. **Medications are chosen based on target symptoms, previous efficacy or adverse response, interactions with other medications, side effect profile, family history of drug response, and cost.**

   a. Children. Because of their smaller size, children have a lower volume of distribution but metabolize drugs at an increased rate. Hence, although children generally require lower doses, the doses tend to be higher in milligrams per kilogram of body weight.

   b. Geriatric patients are more susceptible to adverse side effects and tend to metabolize drugs more slowly. Hence, lower doses are generally used with the elderly.

   c. Medically ill patients are also more sensitive to adverse effects, may have interactions with other medications, and may have increased or decreased rates of metabolism or excretion.

> **HOT**
>
>
>
> **KEY**
>
> The general rule when prescribing psychotropic medications to children, the elderly, or the medically ill is, "Start low, go slow."

   d. Pregnant and nursing patients. Special considerations apply to women who are pregnant or nursing (see Chapter 29).

   e. Dosing considerations. The dose of any psychotropic medication should be increased slowly until an adequate clinical response is seen or side effects occur that prevent further increase. Some psychiatric medications have known **therapeutic levels** that should guide titration. Blood levels will need to be monitored for these agents (see Chapters 16 and 17).

   f. Monitoring. Depending upon the medication and clinical considerations, liver, renal, or thyroid function; blood counts; electrocardiograms; or vital signs may need to be checked at baseline and monitored.

   g. Side effects. The patient must be educated in advance about side effects, and the physician must monitor the patient for them.

   h. Overdose. Many psychiatric medications are toxic in overdose. Overdoses of tricyclic antidepressants and lithium, for example, can be fatal.

HOT **KEY**   For patients who are potentially suicidal, less toxic medications should be chosen, if possible, and prescribed in small amounts to discourage the hoarding of medication and subsequent ingestions.

---

3. Polypharmacy is often used because of psychiatric comorbidities and because of the frequent difficulty in treating symptoms with existing medications.

   a. When prescribing "cocktails" of medications, the medications must be **selected and combined rationally.** For example, adding a medication that increases dopaminergic transmission to one that decreases dopaminergic transmission may not make sense, even if the patient's symptoms fit profiles that may be responsive to each medication.

   b. When using polypharmacy, it is important to consider **potential interactions** with psychiatric and nonpsychiatric medications. Many psychiatric medications are metabolized through the cytochrome P-450 system. Particular classes and medications to be alert to include:

     (1) Antiseizure medications
     (2) Antibiotics
     (3) Antifungal agents
     (4) Cardiac medications (e.g., calcium channel blockers, antiarrhythmic agents, β-blockers)
     (5) Allergy medications
     (6) Hormonal treatments
     (7) Narcotic agents
     (8) Theophylline
     (9) Warfarin sodium
    (10) Omeprazole

      (11) Nicotine

      (12) Caffeine

   c. Simply adding medications to the "cocktail" while losing sight of the "big picture" leads to **malignant polypharmacy,** which results in the patient missing out on appropriate treatment while being exposed to potentially toxic medications.

  4. An adequate medication trial involves a sufficient dose for a sufficient time. Both factors depend upon the patient's clinical state and the particular medication. When a patient does not respond to multiple medication trials, the diagnostic formulation should be revisited. Perhaps the patient is not taking the medication as prescribed, the diagnosis is incorrect, or the symptoms would be better treated via other treatment modalities.

B. Psychological interventions

  1. Psychotherapies are treatments in which verbal interventions are used to modify behavior and ameliorate emotional distress. Most psychotherapy involves a combination of approaches.

   a. Psychoanalysis is aimed at structural reorganization of the personality. It involves four to five sessions per week for psychologically minded, highly motivated, relatively stable individuals. It generally involves focus on early experiences as genetic origins of current symptoms.

   b. Psychodynamic psychotherapy is derived from psychoanalysis; however, it is less intensive, more focused on the present, and has more limited outcomes.

   c. Supportive psychotherapy helps to strengthen ego functions sufficiently so that the individual can cope with everyday demands.

   d. Cognitive therapy is based on the notion that thoughts shape feelings. The goal of cognitive therapy is to change feelings and behaviors by changing the way in which the patient interprets her experiences and views herself.

   e. Behavioral therapy is based on the notion that behaviors are learned. Various techniques are used to change maladaptive behaviors.

   f. Brief psychotherapy involves a variety of techniques, all of which are limited by time and scope of change.

   g. Hypnosis is an approach in which heightened suggestibility is used to affect memory, mood, and perception.

   h. Couples therapy is treatment in the context of the couple and is focused upon the couple's relationship.

   i. Family therapy includes various schools of thought and various approaches, all of which aim to modify family functioning.

      j. Group therapy includes various types of therapeutic groups ranging from psychoeducational to supportive to those that explore interpersonal relationships.

  2. Psychiatric treatment occurs in a **variety of settings.**

      a. The emergency department serves as the point of entry for many patients (see Part II).

      b. Psychiatric inpatient units are generally used to treat people with acute psychiatric disturbances or severe, chronic disturbances. In inpatient settings, the environment itself becomes a therapeutic intervention by providing structure, by modeling behaviors, through peer support, and through the use of token economies.

      c. Partial hospital programs or day hospitals are helpful for patients who require hospital-intensive treatment during the day but can safely return home in the evenings.

      d. Halfway houses can help transition patients from institutions back into the community.

      e. Group homes and residential treatment can provide longer-term interventions.

      f. Intensive **home-based psychiatric services,** in which teams of clinicians provide service directly in the home, can be found in some communities.

      g. Outpatient settings include **clinics** and **private practices.**

C. Social interventions

  1. Social interventions include helping the patient to mobilize family supports, cultivate new supports in the community, minimize external stressors, and access appropriate resources (e.g., medical insurance or housing).

  2. Implementation of social interventions often falls within the domain of **social workers.**

III CASE STUDY–TREATMENT PLAN BASED ON BIOPSYCHOSOCIAL MODEL

A. Formulation. The following treatment plan is based on the patient profile presented in Chapter 2 II C.

B. Treatment plan

  1. Biologic component. Given the strength of the familial predisposition to anxiety and the severity of the patient's symptoms, pharmacological treatment may be considered as part of the treatment plan. An SSRI such as sertraline (Zoloft) would be appropriate. The antianxiety effects may not reach full potential for weeks, and panic symptoms may initially be worsened by the activating side effects of sertraline. Therefore, the patient may initially need to be "covered" by a benzodiazepine such as lorazepam (Ativan) as well.

2. **Psychological component.** The psychological meaning of the symptoms to the patient is adding to his distress and is probably playing a role in driving his symptoms; therefore, psychotherapy should be considered for this patient. Psychodynamic psychotherapy may be appropriate. When the unconscious conflicts underlying his symptoms are made conscious, he will have more control and less need to express his feelings somatically.

3. **Social component.** The patient's history of stressors includes social deprivation and exposure to multiple traumas. The treatment plan may include further assessment of the patient's environment, family functioning, and current access to appropriate services. This aspect of the treatment plan may involve enlisting the services of a social worker.

References

*Baxter LR Jr, Schwartz JM, Bergman KS, et al: Caudate glucose metabolic rate changes with both drug and behavior therapy for obsessive–compulsive disorder. *Arch Gen Psychiatry* 49:681, 1992.

Cramer JA, Rosenheck R: Compliance with medication regimens for mental and physical disorders. *Psychiatr Serv* 49(2):196–201, 1998.

*classic reference

5. Psychological Assessment

I **INTRODUCTION.** Psychological assessment tools provide a structured way to obtain information regarding a patient's capacities and behaviors.

A. **Psychological testing** covers a variety of areas, including:
—Intellectual ability
—Academic achievement
—Adaptive behavior
—Personality functioning

B. **Neuropsychological evaluations** assess brain–behavior relationships. Such assessments may include measures of sensory perceptual functions, motor functions, psychomotor problem solving, language and communication skills, and other cognitive and intellectual capacities. Neuropsychological testing is useful for such functions as differentiating brain-damaged patients from those who are not brain damaged; localizing hemispheric involvement; differentiating static from rapidly growing lesions; and planning for rehabilitation. This chapter focuses on psychological, rather than neuropsychological, testing.

II **APPROACH TO THE PATIENT**

A. **Referral questions.** To maximize its clinical usefulness, the testing should be directed toward answering specific referral questions. For example, the referring physician for a patient who is having trouble concentrating might want to know whether a patient's difficulties reflect attentional problems or emotional problems, such as depression. Appropriate referral questions facilitate the clinician's choice of test instruments and interpretation of relevant issues. Referral questions are often formulated by the referring doctor. If the referring doctor is uncertain about the goals of testing, consultation with the testing clinician can help focus referral questions.

B. **Preparation of patients.** In order for psychological testing to be most useful, the patient should be told in clear, nontechnical language what to expect from the testing and why it is being administered. Generally, the preparation is initiated by the referring doctor and completed by the testing clinician.

III TEST ADMINISTRATION

A. Battery composition. After the referral question is clarified, the examiner must decide which instruments to use. **Test battery** refers to the group of tests chosen for a particular patient.

   1. In making this determination, the evaluator must balance the desire to obtain a maximum amount of data against such practical factors as the need for expeditious completion of the evaluation and the patient's capacity to tolerate the rigors of testing.

   2. The evaluator will also consider adjusting the battery composition as emerging test data refine the referral question or suggest new questions.

B. Length of administration. The length of time required for a patient to complete a test battery depends upon a number of factors, including the complexity of the referral question, the associated number of test instruments, and the patient's capacity for sustained work on focused tasks.

HOT KEY The administration of a comprehensive psychological assessment battery usually requires four to six sessions of approximately 60–90 minutes each.

C. Obtaining the patient's best efforts. Because the goal of testing generally is to obtain a picture of the patient's maximum capacities, the clinician must develop sufficient rapport to ensure the patient's best efforts. The examiner employs clinical skills to allay the patient's anxiety and enlist cooperation in completing the tasks at hand.

HOT KEY The examiner must be certain that the establishment of rapport does not interfere with the administration of tests according to standardized procedures.

IV COMMONLY USED ASSESSMENT INSTRUMENTS

A. Measures of intellectual ability

   1. Wechsler Adult Intelligence Scale–Third Edition (WAIS-III). The WAIS-III assumes that intelligence is defined as an individual's capacity to understand and cope with the world. The WAIS-III may be used with patients between the ages of 16 years and 74 years and 11 months.

2. **Wechsler Intelligence Scale for Children–Third Edition (WISC-III).** The WISC-III is a downward extension of the WAIS and is designed for children ranging in age from 6 years to 16 years and 11 months.

3. **Kaufman Adolescent and Adult Intelligence Test (KAIT).** The KAIT measures novel problem-solving skills **(fluid intelligence)** and knowledge derived from acculturation and education **(crystallized intelligence).** A core battery can be administered in less than an hour and can be used for individuals from 11 to 85 years of age.

4. **Stanford-Binet, 4th Edition (SB:FE).**
   a. The SB:FE is based on a three-level theoretical model of intelligence:
      (1) a general intelligence factor at the highest level
      (2) a second level that includes crystallized intelligence, fluid intelligence, and short-term memory
      (3) a final level including such factors as verbal, quantitative, and abstract visual reasoning
   b. The SB:FE is used for individuals from 2 to 23 years of age.

B. **Measures of academic achievement**
   1. **Wide Range Achievement Test–Third Edition (WRAT-III).** The WRAT has been used for many years as a brief screener to identify academic skills and deficits. It is designed for individuals from 5 to 75 years of age.
   2. **Kaufman Test of Educational Achievement (K-TEA).** The K-TEA assesses academic achievement in children from 5 to 18 years of age.
   3. **Woodcock Johnson Tests of Achievement (WJ).** The WJ estimates level of scholastic accomplishments for kindergarten through 12th grade.

C. **Measures of adaptive behavior**
   —**Vineland Adaptive Behavior Scales.** This interview assesses an individual's personal and social sufficiency. It can be used to evaluate the adaptive functioning of mentally retarded individuals of all ages and nonretarded individuals up to 19 years of age.

D. **Projective tests.** Projective tests generally present patients with ambiguous or incomplete stimuli (e.g., pictures or inkblots) on which the patient projects his own unconscious concerns, often revealing aspects of his inner life.
   1. **Rorschach inkblots.** The Rorschach, consisting of 10 inkblots, is primarily used to assess personality organization. It evaluates such issues as the patient's capacity for reality testing, integration of affect, and human relations. The Exner scoring system is one method for scoring the Rorschach.

2. **Thematic Apperception Test (TAT).** The TAT consists of picture cards about which the patient is asked to tell a story.
3. **Projective drawings.** In projective drawing tasks, including Draw-A-Person, House-Tree-Person, and Kinetic Family, the patient's drawings, produced under standardized procedures, are subjected to a qualitative analysis, revealing such data as the patient's view of his self, social environment, and family relations.

E. **Personality tests**
   —Minnesota Multiphasic Personality Inventory (MMPI). The MMPI consists of nearly 500 true–false items completed by the patient. The MMPI produces a patient profile based on various scales (e.g., depression, paranoia, hypochondria, anger, bizarre mentation, alcoholism).

 PSYCHOLOGICAL TEST RESULTS. Some general concerns must be kept in mind when assessing the results of any psychological test battery.

A. **Interpretation of findings.** For each area evaluated (e.g., cognition or personality), test findings place the patient at a particular level of functioning. However, it is important to understand the profile of strengths and weaknesses within each area and to analyze how the separate areas relate to each other. Ultimately, psychological assessment should provide a well-integrated, comprehensive view of the patient.

B. **Communication of findings.** Test results should first be communicated to the referring doctor. The examiner and referring doctor should then decide how best to communicate the test findings to the patient and, where appropriate, to the patient's family. In any event, test results should be explained in understandable language and with sensitivity. Test findings are best accepted and understood in the context of a supportive, therapeutic relationship.

Reference
Halperin JM, McKay KE: Psychological testing for psychiatrists. *J Am Acad Child Adolesc Psychiatry* 37:575–584, 1998.

PART II

EMERGENCY PSYCHIATRY

6. Assessment in the Emergency Department

I. INITIAL EVALUATION

A. Team approach. Effective evaluation of a patient in crisis requires a team approach. If you are seeing a patient for the first time in an emergency department (ED) setting, keep in mind that the help of other staff members is vital for adding information to your own clinical assessment and helping you manage the patient. Family or significant others should be interviewed. Police should be interviewed, if they are involved.

B. Formulation of a treatment plan. Most patient evaluations in the ED are targeted at crisis intervention and initiating a plan for more comprehensive assessment and treatment. In order to formulate a treatment plan for any patient, you need to address the following questions:

1. Is the patient acutely agitated and in need of immediate treatment?

2. Is the patient's presentation due to underlying toxic or medical causes?

3. Is the patient likely to hurt himself or others?

4. Is the patient capable of self-care?

 HOT KEY Because many patients are quite volatile and may be aggressive, you must not only protect the patient but also keep your own safety in mind when working in an ED setting.

C. Safety. The question **"How safe am I with this patient?"** should be considered before the interview is begun. If the patient is extremely paranoid or acutely agitated, you should be especially careful. However, it is important to realize that an outwardly calm patient may become violent without apparent warning in the case of severe underlying mental illness. Universal precautions must be taken when approaching any patient for the first time.

1. **Assume nothing.**
2. **Maintain your awareness of the environment and potential hazards** (e.g., sharp objects) **at all times.**

HOT KEY

You should never be in a location where the patient could corner you or where other staff would not hear you if you needed help.

---

3. **Have the patient searched for weapons** if there is any question of concealed arms.
4. **Use as quiet an area as possible,** to reduce distracting or aggravating stimuli.
5. **Position yourself,** not the patient, **near the door** in case the patient becomes agitated and you need to leave the area.
6. **Do not touch the patient** (other than to shake hands if appropriate).
7. **Maintain a calm and respectful demeanor** to help the patient to stay in control.
8. End the interview, leave the area, and ask for staff **assistance if the patient becomes agitated.**

D. **Assaultive behavior and the agitated patient.** It is not uncommon to have a patient present to the ED in an extremely agitated state. The evaluation of such a patient is clearly more urgent, but the most important initial step is to make sure the patient and staff are safe.
   1. **Try to identify what, if anything, is fueling the patient's agitation.** Sometimes if you can identify the source of agitation (e.g., another patient or a family member accompanying the patient), you can diffuse the situation.
   2. **Offer the patient some time in a quiet area to help him calm down.** Talk gently but firmly to the patient about his need to stay in behavioral control.
   3. **Medications may be necessary to help calm an agitated patient if other interventions fail.** Offer medications by mouth, but if they are refused, tell the patient that she will be given the drug intramuscularly if her behavior remains extreme. A rapid assessment of the patient will help guide your decision about when to use medications and which ones to use.
      a. A high-potency antipsychotic should be used when psychotic symptoms are evident (e.g., droperidol, 2 to 5 mg intramuscularly, or haloperidol [Haldol], 5 mg by mouth or intramuscularly). To offset the possibility of a dystonic

reaction, diphenhydramine (Benadryl), 50 mg by mouth or intramuscularly, can be coadministered with it.

    b. If the patient is anxious, distraught, and combative or out of control, a better choice may be lorazepam (Ativan), 2 mg by mouth or intramuscularly.

4. Never attempt to restrain the patient yourself. ED staff are trained to know how and when to use restraints for safety. Unless you have been trained yourself in how to place a patient in restraints, resist the urge to help because you could be injured.

5. Consider what role alcohol, drug, or metabolic toxicity could be playing in the patient's condition.

6. Once the patient is calm and in better control, reassess him clinically.

II   APPROACH TO THE PATIENT

A. Medical work-up

    1. The second most important question (after safety) is **"Is there an underlying medical cause for the patient's presentation?"** This is vital to the patient because some conditions may be life-threatening if not treated promptly. All patients who present for evaluation in the ED should have an appropriate medical work-up. For most patients, this should include:

        a. Physical examination, including neurological assessment and vital signs

        b. Chest radiograph if not done in the past 12 months

        c. Electrocardiogram

        d. Urinalysis

        e. Laboratory tests

            (1) Electrolytes

            (2) Liver enzyme tests

            (3) Complete blood count (CBC) with differential

        f. Thyroid function studies

        g. Toxicology screen (for alcohol, opiates, cocaine, and benzodiazepines)

        h. Pregnancy test (for women of child-bearing age)

        i. Consider computed tomography of head or lumbar puncture

    2. Follow good clinical judgment in adding other tests as necessary. For instance, include serum acetaminophen, salicylate, and tricyclic antidepressant levels on any patient suspected of ingesting pills in a suicide attempt. Not all tests need to be repeated if the patient presents to the ED frequently. Request old medical records, which will help to identify the patient's past psychiatric and medical disorders and medications that have been used.

    3. A number of **medical illnesses may cause psychiatric symptoms** (see **Table 6-1**).

TABLE 6-1. Medical Conditions and Associated Psychiatric and Physical Manifestations

Medical Condition	Associated Psychiatric Manifestations	Associated Physical Manifestations
Hyperthyroidism	Irritability, insomnia, anxiety, pressured speech, panic	Tachycardia, heat intolerance, sweating, diarrhea, tremor
Hypothyroidism	Lethargy, depressed mood, paranoia or psychosis	Psychomotor slowing, muscle weakness, dry skin, constipation, goiter, cold intolerance
Hyperglycemia	Anxiety, agitation	Polyuria, increased thirst and dehydration, anorexia
Hypoglycemia	Anxiety, confusion	Sweating, nausea, drowsiness or stupor
Brain neoplasm or injury	Personality changes, mood lability, impaired judgment, confusion, memory impairment, hallucinations	Seizures, neurologic deficits
AIDS	Progressive dementia, depressed mood, psychosis	Fever, weight loss, seizures, incontinence
Hyponatremia	Confusion, lethargy, personality changes	Polydipsia, seizures, speech abnormalities
Systemic lupus erythematosus	Mood disturbances, psychosis, hallucinations	Fever, butterfly rash, joint pain, headache
Multiple sclerosis	Anxiety, euphoria, depression	Focal motor or sensory deficits, incontinence, visual impairment
Hepatic encephalopathy	Lethargy, confusion, disinhibition, psychosis	Asterixis, ataxia, liver enlargement or atrophy, ecchymoses, angiomata
Acute intermittent porphyria	Acute depression, agitation, paranoia	Abdominal pain, nausea, vomiting leukocytosis, paralysis, neuropathy

(*continued*)

TABLE 6-1. Medical Conditions and Associated Psychiatric and Physical Manifestations (*Continued*)

Medical Condition	Associated Psychiatric Manifestations	Associated Physical Manifestations
Thiamine deficiency	Confusion, amnesia, confabulation	Nystagmus, headache, cardiomyopathy, neuropathy
Seizure disorder	Confusion, lethargy, personality changes, bizarre repetitive behavior	Staring spells, tonic–clonic movements, transient motor or language deficits
B_{12} deficiency	Dementia, inattentiveness, psychosis	Ataxia, fatigue, pallor, megaloblastic anemia

AIDS = acquired immune deficiency syndrome.

4. The **chronically mentally ill often have poor or no medical care** and as a result suffer from conditions such as uncontrolled hypertension, anemia due to chronic lice infestation, malnutrition, and other problems.

B. Psychiatric assessment. Although getting a detailed clinical history may be hampered by the patient's mental status, every psychiatric assessment includes a formal evaluation of the patient. Your goal is to obtain the following information during your assessment of a patient in the ED:

1. **Mental status examination (see also Chapter 3).** A mental status examination is the examiner's fundamental tool in the emergency setting.

   a. The **patient's appearance and level of cooperativity** should be described as accurately as possible.

   b. The presence of any **abnormalities in thought process** should be carefully assessed (e.g., disorganization).

   c. Any **thoughts of suicide** or **urges to hurt others** should be fully explored (see Chapter 7).

   d. **Formal cognitive testing**—orientation, memory, and abstraction testing—should be included as it can often help identify psychotic or cognitively impaired patients.

   e. The patient's insight and judgment skills should be tested regarding issues of **self-care,** their mental illness, and plans to cope with their current situation if discharged.

2. Patient history. There is much to be learned from careful observation of a patient, even one who is incoherent or refuses to be interviewed. Begin by describing how the patient came to the ED (e.g., did she walk in, was she brought in by emergency medical services?). You may need to interview family members or friends who can provide collateral history for the patient, especially if there is any question about the patient's safety.

  a. Previous psychiatric illness should be noted, including:
    (1) The presenting symptoms and medications used
    (2) The number of hospitalizations and precipitating factors
    (3) The degree of compliance with recommended treatments

  b. Substance abuse history should be noted, including:
    (1) Substances used, how often, and whether the patient sees it as a problem
    (2) If the patient was treated for substance abuse, how long he remained sober afterward

  c. Brief personal and social history should be noted, including:
    (1) How he spends his time now—work, social life, leisure time—and where he lives
    (2) Friends or other family members with whom she maintains contact for support
    (3) Education, military, and employment history will tell you about the patient's ability to function in the past.

  d. Medical history. Learn the patient's medical history, current medical problems, and medications.

References

Ghaemi SN, Pope HG Jr: Lack of insight in psychotic and affective disorders: A review of empirical studies. *Harv Rev Psychiatry* 2(1):22–33, 1994.

Knopp RK, Satterlee PA: Confidentiality in the emergency department. *Emerg Med Clin North Am* 17(2):385–396, 1999.

7. Suicide

I **INTRODUCTION.** The **most frequent psychiatric complaints** in the emergency department (ED) are **suicide attempts** and **suicidal ideation.**

A. Suicidal ideation can be prompted by **any stressor that becomes overwhelming** to the patient and fuels the **desire to escape.** The stressor is usually a loss.

B. The physician must **determine how serious the risk of suicide** is for a particular patient and **what steps to take** to ensure a patient can remain safe.

II **CLINICAL MANIFESTATIONS**

A. Suicide attempts
1. **Drug overdose** is probably the most frequent means of suicide attempt seen in the ED. People who attempt suicide by more violent means (e.g., shooting a gun, jumping off a building, hanging) are generally more successful—you don't see these patients.
2. Many people who attempt suicide and fail are engaging in **"suicide gestures"**—self-destructive behavior that is meant to be nonlethal.
   a. These patients may take drug overdoses or cut or burn themselves superficially and then tell someone what they've done.
   b. These patients often have underlying problems with impulsivity and mood regulation as a result of a personality disorder or are acting in response to psychotic thought content.

B. Suicidal ideation is the contemplation of a desire to die or to take steps toward killing oneself.
1. A complaint of suicidal ideation can take a variety of forms, such as:
   a. "It's just not worth it anymore."
   b. "I have a gun and almost used it."
2. Sometimes a patient is brought to medical attention by a relative or friend who suspects he wants to kill himself:
   a. The person may have **threatened** to do so.
   b. The person may have been **depressed, withdrawn,** or **acting strangely.**
3. Patients who present with suicidal ideation may be:
   a. **Intoxicated**

  b. In a state of **withdrawal from drugs or alcohol**
  c. In the **midst of a crisis such as a divorce or separation**

III CAUSES

A. The **trigger for acting** on a suicidal impulse may vary but most
often it is **feeling truly hopeless** about one's situation and de-
ciding there is "no way out."

B. There may be **biologic risk factors** that make some people vulnerable to suicide attempts, independent of their psychiatric illness. The threshold for suicidal behavior appears to be lower in
individuals with lower serotonergic function.

C. There are a number of **risk factors** that increase the likelihood
that a suicide attempt will be made.

  1. **Patients with mood disorders** comprise 80% of people who
  attempt suicide.

  2. A history of **alcohol abuse** is present in 25% of people who
  attempt suicide.

  3. Approximately 10% of patients with **schizophrenia** commit
  suicide.

  4. The mnemonic "SUICIDAL" will help you remember the
  most important risk factors for suicide:

Risk Factors for Suicide ("SUICIDAL")

Social withdrawal
Utter hopelessness or helplessness
Insomnia
Chronic physical illness or pain
Impulsivity or previous suicide attempts
Drug abuse or alcoholism
Alone or socially isolated
Loss of interpersonal relationship

IV APPROACH TO THE PATIENT

A. If the potential for suicide is a concern, **make sure that the patient is not left alone** and that any **potentially dangerous objects
have been removed** from the room.

B. There is no truth to the idea that talking about suicide will induce a patient to try it. **You must ask the patient about suicide
directly** in every assessment you make. Use the following guidelines to explore the patient's suicidal ideation:

  1. Begin by asking her about **feelings of hopelessness, worthlessness,** or the desire to "never wake up again."

  2. What **specific thoughts** has she had about wanting to kill herself?

    a. Does she have a **plan** in mind to kill herself?
    b. How frequently do the thoughts occur? Has it been **increasingly frequent?**
  3. Does she have **access to the means** of killing herself if she has a plan?
  4. If so, **how close to acting** on this plan has she come so far?
  5. Has she **tried to confide in anyone** about her thoughts?
  6. Is there **anyone she could talk to?**
  7. Can she **imagine any way in which things could get better?**
C. If the patient has already made an attempt, also ask:
  1. Was the suicide attempt impulsive, or did he plan it in any way?
  2. How lethal did he think his attempt was likely to be?
  3. How did he come to be saved? (Was he discovered or did he ask for help?)
  4. What is his feeling about still being alive?
  5. Does he have any continued suicidal ideation?
D. Finally, if a patient is being uncooperative, **interview significant others** to obtain as much history as possible. Ask about mood symptoms they may have noticed or any strange behavior, such as giving away his possessions or saying good-bye in other ways.

HOT **KEY**   Often a patient will report suicidal ideation to avoid going to jail if legal issues are at hand. These reports must be taken seriously, however, and precautions taken. Many jails have observation cells for such patients.

V   **EVALUATING RISK.** While there is no foolproof way of predicting whether someone is likely to commit suicide, any of the following should alert you to the need to get urgent treatment for the patient:

A. Recent major loss or continued, unresolved stressor
B. Depressed mood with hopelessness
C. Lack of social support
D. Recent suicide attempt
  1. If the attempt was made impulsively in the throes of a crisis and the patient is relieved she did not die, she is more likely to be safe now.
  2. If the patient or significant others describe a weeks- or months-long trend toward despair and a process of letting go of friends and possessions, the patient needs careful monitoring and probably hospitalization.
E. Patients who have been depressed with extreme psychomotor retardation **and who are becoming more animated** but are still depressed **are at high risk because now they have the energy to act** on suicidal impulses.
F. Patients with psychotic disorders or **patients who are under the**

influence of drugs or alcohol must be taken seriously when they express suicidal ideation because they are much more likely to act on suicidal thoughts and to use methods of high lethality.

VI **TREATMENT.** If you decide a patient is at significant risk of suicide, he may still be treated in the outpatient setting if he can reliably contract for safety, with the help of his friends or family.

A. Begin **antidepressant treatment** and substance abuse treatment as appropriate.

B. **Hospitalize** the patient, even involuntarily, if you cannot be sure of the patient's ability to follow through with treatment, or you distrust his reliability.

   1. Sometimes patients will require long-term hospitalization until significant mood changes can be effected through medication or electroconvulsive therapy.

   2. Patients may benefit from short-term hospital stays, especially in the event of a crisis, or when their own impulsivity needs containment.

   3. Because suicide gestures can sometimes turn into completed attempts, it is often helpful to briefly hospitalize patients who have a recurrent pattern of suicide attempts.

VII **FOLLOW-UP AND REFERRAL.** If a patient is at low but still significant risk for suicide and you are planning to discharge him from the ED, you must have a follow-up plan in place.

A. Give the patient specific instructions in writing about where to go for treatment, with a name and phone number of a clinician to contact. Reiterate the instructions to family members or significant others who can continue to provide support after the patient leaves the ED.

B. If a new medication is being prescribed, explain the possible side effects and the need to continue treatment as prescribed, even if the benefits are not evident (e.g., some antidepressants may not show effects for 2–4 weeks).

C. Remind both the patient and family that the patient should return to the ED if thoughts of suicide return and become overwhelming or if there is any question about her ability to remain safe.

D. Document the referral instructions and follow-up plan items.

References

Hall RC, Platt DE, Hall RC: Suicide risk assessment: A review of risk factors for suicide in 100 patients who made severe suicide attempts. Evaluation of suicide risk in a time of managed care. *Psychosomatics* 40(1):18–27, 1999.

Mann JJ, Oquendo M, Underwood MD, Arango V: The neurobiology of suicide risk: A review for the clinician. *J Clin Psychiatry* 60(suppl 2):7–11; discussion 18–20, 113–116, 1999.

Prudic J, Sackheim HA: Electroconvulsive therapy and suicide risk. *J Clin Psychiatry* 60(suppl 2):104–110; discussion 111–116, 1999.

8. Generating a Disposition in the Emergency Setting

I INTRODUCTION

A. **Emergency disposition.** The goal of treatment in the emergency department (ED) is to identify clinical problems and begin the appropriate treatment. The next phase of treatment involves disposition. This usually entails one of the following:
   1. Admitting the patient to a psychiatric or medical service
   2. Discharging the patient to outpatient services
   3. Detaining the patient for a short-term stay in the ED (i.e., 24–72 hours), during which more prolonged assessment or crisis intervention may be done
B. **Developing a plan.** To develop a plan—a disposition—you will need to:
   1. Understand the patient's clinical status, support system, and living situation
   2. Recommend appropriate services that are available
C. **Gathering patient information for disposition**
   1. The patient must get **medical clearance** for discharge, and you must complete your **psychiatric assessment.**
   2. **Try to contact a family member or friend** to help answer any questions that still remain about the patient's history or current situation that would guide your treatment.
   3. **Make a treatment decision** based on your clinical understanding of the patient.

II IS THE PATIENT SAFE TO DISCHARGE? There are four key questions you should use to assess whether the patient is safe to discharge:

A. **Ability to remain in control**—has the patient been able to wait in the ED setting without her condition escalating? Does the patient have any past history of impulsivity when faced with stressful situations? If a patient is very agitated, hospitalization is usually warranted, even if involuntary.
B. **Medical problems or toxic exposure**—have these been ruled out as possible causes of the patient's condition? If not, are they able to be addressed on an outpatient basis? Any medically unstable patients (including patients in withdrawal from alcohol) need to be admitted for treatment.

C. Suicidal or homicidal ideation—if the patient has thoughts of harm to self or others or has made an actual attempt, you must not discharge a patient unless:

1. He can reliably contract for safety (see Chapter 7).

2. The patient's history suggests he will comply with follow-up.

3. A family member or friend can corroborate the patient's history and offer support in case the harmful thoughts or feelings increase in intensity.

HOT

In general, a patient who has attempted to harm himself or others must be admitted for evaluation and treatment.

KEY

D. Self-care—generally, patients with gross cognitive impairment or severe mood or psychotic symptoms are unable to manage the day-to-day requirements for living (e.g., obtaining food, water, and safe shelter).

1. Patients unable to care for themselves always warrant hospitalization, and if the condition is chronic, long-term care will need to be arranged.

2. If a patient refuses hospitalization, involuntary hospitalization may be allowed (see section III) to maintain patient safety in the face of self-neglect.

III INVOLUNTARY HOSPITALIZATION

A. Hospitalization of a patient over her objections is permitted if the right conditions are met.

1. You must offer a patient voluntary hospitalization first.

2. If a patient does not want to be hospitalized, but you feel she is a danger to herself—either because of the risk of suicide or self-neglect—or a danger to others, you may hospitalize her involuntarily.

B. State laws vary in the requirements for additional assessments to corroborate your clinical assessment.

1. In some states, involuntary hospitalization on an emergency basis only requires one physician, but a second physician must agree with this decision to extend the admission beyond 24 or 72 hours.

2. At any time, a patient may request discharge, which forces a legal hearing in which a judge will make the final determination.

IV OUTPATIENT DISPOSITIONS

A. Referral to outpatient treatment. If you have decided that a patient may be discharged, a referral to outpatient treatment with a psychiatrist is usually appropriate.

1. Your role as the clinician responsible for the patient's care in the current crisis also involves helping to form a plan for follow-up.
2. Follow-up treatment can help avert a similar crisis in the future.

B. Outpatient services. Being familiar with available services for continued outpatient treatment is enormously helpful in the ED. Many EDs have social work support staff that are adept at directing a patient to appropriate clinics or programs. The types of outpatient services most frequently needed are:

1. Psychiatric clinics for psychotherapy and psychotropic medication management
2. Substance abuse treatment centers—for detoxification or rehabilitation from drugs and alcohol
3. Support groups (e.g., domestic violence support groups, Alcoholics Anonymous, Narcotics Anonymous, Gamblers Anonymous)
4. Partial hospital programs
5. Social services—for benefits (e.g., welfare, Medicaid, housing, food stamps)

V DOCUMENTATION.

There are several important reasons to carefully document your full clinical assessment of the patient and your interactions in the ED.

A. A **patient's mental status** upon presenting to the ED **may change from hour to hour or even minute to minute.** As the evaluation proceeds, an accurate assessment depends upon a complete clinical picture as evidenced in the medical record.

B. Other people will usually be taking over the care of the patient you are seeing now, and your careful summaries will be invaluable guides to their understanding of the treatment issues. For instance, if a patient arrives at the ED malodorous, unkempt, and incoherent, the need for psychosocial intervention will be obvious. Three days later, with a shower and some medication, the same patient may not appear to others to be as disorganized, and those involved with follow-up treatment may underestimate the patient's needs, especially if the patient has impaired insight into her own illness.

C. The **need for involuntary hospitalization must always be outlined** because this is a legal deprivation of the patient's right to self-determination. The appropriate use of involuntary hospitalization is important to good clinical care, but you must fully inform others by documenting your reasoning.

D. Sometimes a patient will attempt to sue the institution or practitioners for alleged acts of malpractice or other abuse. A clear record of all interactions is the best defense in legal cases. Make sure to document any evidence of antisocial behavior, refusal to follow recommended treatment, as well as your clinical interventions.

HOT KEY — Documentation should include telling the patient to return to the ED as needed or if symptoms worsen.

References

Atakan Z, Davies T: ABC of mental health. Mental health emergencies. *BMJ* 314(7096):1740–1742, 1997.

Lidz CW, Hoge SK, Gardner W, et al: Perceived coercion in mental hospital admission. Pressures and process. *Arch Gen Psychiatry* 52(12):1034–1039, 1995.

Wettstein RM: The right to refuse psychiatric treatment. *Psychiatr Clin North Am* 22(1):173–182, viii, 1999.

PART III

PSYCHOTIC DISORDERS

9. Overview of Psychosis

I **INTRODUCTION.** The phenomenon of psychosis may be present in a variety of psychiatric and medical disorders.

A. There are various definitions of the term **psychosis.**
  1. The hallmark, however, is generally considered to be **impaired reality testing,** which is the inability to distinguish between what is real and what is not real.
  2. A broader definition is based on the **presence** of any of a number of **characteristic symptoms,** including hallucinations, delusions, disorganized speech, and disorganized or catatonic behavior.
B. This chapter provides a general overview of psychosis. The next two chapters discuss schizophrenia—the prototypical psychotic disorder—and antipsychotic treatment.

II **CAUSES.** Psychosis may be seen in a great variety of medical and psychiatric conditions. Because there are many specific causes, it is useful to divide them into the broad categories of primary psychiatric disorders, medical conditions, substance-induced conditions, and psychotic disorder not otherwise specified (NOS).

A. **Primary psychiatric disorders** include psychoses without a known physiologic or anatomic cause that are considered to have a psychiatric cause.
B. **Medical conditions** can cause patients to present with psychoses resulting from central nervous system dysfunction caused by known organic factors (e.g., stroke, infection, trauma, tumor). This category as presented here includes dementia and delirium because these can often be related to a known organic cause.
C. **Substance-induced psychoses** are caused by the direct effects of ingestion of a substance.
D. **Psychotic disorder NOS** is a category of psychoses for which not enough information is known to infer a cause.

III CLINICAL MANIFESTATIONS OF PSYCHOSIS

A. Primary psychiatric disorders include a spectrum of psychiatric illnesses in which psychosis may be seen. Some patients with psychiatric illnesses present with psychosis as a defining feature (e.g., schizophrenia) and some psychiatric illnesses are primarily nonpsychotic but when severe, or when the patient is under stress, psychotic symptoms may be present (e.g., in major depression or personality disorders).

1. **Schizophrenia** is a chronic illness that lasts a minimum of 6 months and is characterized by exacerbations and remissions. It is also associated with marked social or occupational impairment. The acute psychotic episodes are marked by delusions, hallucinations, disorganized speech, bizarre behavior, or flattened or inappropriate affect (see Chapter 10).

2. **Schizophreniform disorder** is characterized by the same features as **schizophrenia** except the total duration of the illness is at least 1 month but less than 6 months, and there may not be impaired social or occupational functioning.

3. **Schizoaffective disorder** is a disease that combines features of **schizophrenia** with those of a **mood disorder** (see Chapters 15 and 17). During the course of the illness there is a manic, depressed, or mixed episode that includes psychotic symptoms. There is also a period of the illness in which there are hallucinations or delusions without mood symptoms.

4. **Delusional disorder** is an illness that lasts for at least 1 month and is marked by the presence of one or more nonbizarre (not impossible) delusions. Auditory hallucinations are not prominent.

5. **Brief psychotic disorder** has the sudden onset of delusions, hallucinations, disorganized speech, or bizarre behavior. It lasts at least 1 day but less than a month.

6. Patients with **mood disorders,** specifically **manic episodes** and **major depression,** can present with psychotic features during severe episodes.

7. Patients with **personality disorders,** especially **schizotypal, schizoid, borderline,** and **paranoid,** can present with psychotic symptoms.

HOT KEY   When people with personality disorders are under stress, they may develop brief episodes of psychosis lasting minutes to hours.

B. Medical conditions that can cause symptoms of psychosis comprise a vast array of illnesses. These can be divided into the diagnoses of **psychotic disorder due to a general medical condition, dementia,** and **delirium.** Unlike primary psychiatric disorders, these diagnoses have a potentially known organic cause that may be treatable.

1. **Psychotic disorder due to a general medical condition** is a diagnosis made when there is evidence from the history, physical examination, or laboratory studies that the symptoms (e.g., hallucinations or delusions) are due to the physiologic effects of a general medical condition. This diagnosis is not made if the symptoms occur during the course of a **delirium** or a **dementia.**

HOT

KEY

Medical conditions that can result in psychosis include neoplasms, epilepsy, stroke, head trauma, AIDS, neurosyphilis, Wilson's disease, and systemic lupus erythematosus (SLE).

---

2. **Dementia,** although the defining characteristics are multiple cognitive deficits including memory impairment, can also include psychotic symptoms (see Chapter 46). Common psychotic symptoms seen in patients with dementia include persecutory delusions (e.g., the belief that personal items are being stolen) and hallucinations, especially visual hallucinations or atypical auditory hallucinations (e.g., hearing music).

3. **Delirium** is marked by the acute onset of disturbances in consciousness and attention that fluctuate during the course of a day. There may be vivid hallucinations, delusions, and disorganized speech. Compared with those found in the psychotic disorders, the psychotic symptoms of delirium are more likely to fluctuate and to vary in nature during the course of a delirium (see Chapter 25).

HOT

KEY

Delirium tends to be reversible, unlike most dementias.

C. **Substance-induced** psychotic symptoms are the direct effects of a substance. A variety of substances can cause psychosis either due to exposure or to withdrawal. The diagnosis of **substance-induced psychotic disorder** is made only if there is impaired reality testing (i.e., the patient believes that the hallucination or delusion is real and does not recognize that it is caused by a substance). If reality testing is intact, the diagnosis may be simply **substance intoxication** or **substance withdrawal.**

1. **Medications used for a variety of conditions can cause psychosis.** These include **anesthetics, anticholinergics, antihypertensives, antibiotics, antiparkinsonian agents, chemotherapy agents, corticosteroids,** and **over-the-counter medications.**

2. **Toxins** that can cause psychosis include certain insecticides, carbon monoxide, some types of paint, and heavy metals.

3. **Intoxication** with alcohol and illicit drugs, including amphetamines, cannabis, cocaine, hallucinogens, inhalants, opioids, and phencyclidine (PCP), can cause psychotic symptoms that vary with the substance. For example, cocaine and amphetamine intoxication can present with persecutory delusions or tactile hallucinations. Generally, the psychosis resolves after the period of intoxication, but the symptoms can last weeks or longer.

4. **Withdrawal** from alcohol, sedatives, hypnotics, and anxiolytics can cause psychotic symptoms. Depending on the substance involved, symptoms can develop anywhere from hours to weeks after cessation of use.

D. **Psychotic disorder NOS** includes disturbances with psychotic symptoms that do not meet the criteria for any other specific disorder or when there is not enough information available to make any other diagnosis. This diagnosis can be made if psychotic symptoms are present but it cannot be determined if they are primary, are due to a medical condition, or are substance induced.

IV APPROACH TO THE PATIENT

A. The **mental status examination** (see Chapter 3) is important for assessing the presence and nature of psychotic symptoms as well as their stability or fluctuation over time. This is crucial for establishing the diagnosis. Special attention should be paid to **speech, mood, affect, thought process,** and **thought content.**

B. The **patient history** is also crucial for making a diagnosis because the disorders have varying patterns in terms of time course, exacerbations and remissions, and relationship to physical symptoms or substance use. Special attention should be paid to the **prodromal symptoms, onset and duration of symptoms, history of similar symptoms, prescribed medications,** and **substance use.** A **family history** of psychiatric symptoms should also be obtained.

C. A **physical examination** and **laboratory studies** are necessary to evaluate for the possibility of an underlying medical condition or substance abuse. Special attention should be paid to the **neurologic examination** and to the **electrolyte and glucose levels, liver function test, thyroid function test, rapid plasmin reagin test (RPR),** and **toxicology** and **illicit drug screen.** In cases in which dementia is suspected, **B₁₂** and **folate levels** should be obtained. In cases of new-onset psychosis with no evidence of substance use, a **computed tomography (CT) scan of the head** should be considered to rule out a brain neoplasm or other structural abnormality. **Electroencephalography (EEG)** should be considered if seizures are suggested by the history.

 V TREATMENT AND FOLLOW-UP depend on the cause of the psychosis. Patients with medical conditions causing psychosis should be evaluated by an internist to treat the underlying pathology. Management of a patient with a primary psychiatric disorder, a substance-induced disorder, or psychosis NOS depends on the nature of the psychiatric symptoms and their cause (see Chapters 10 and 11).

References

Crespo-Facorro B, Piven ML, Schultz SK: Psychosis in late life: How does it fit into current diagnostic criteria? *Am J Psychiatry* 156:624–629, 1999.

Franzek E, Beckmann H: Different genetic background of schizophrenia spectrum psychoses: A twin study. *Am J Psychiatry* 155:76–83, 1998.

10. Schizophrenia

I INTRODUCTION. Schizophrenia is a chronic illness that can be devastating to many aspects of a patient's life. It is characterized by **hallucinations, delusions, behavioral disturbances, and disrupted social and occupational functioning.** About 10% of patients with schizophrenia commit suicide. The lifetime prevalence of schizophrenia is about 1%.

HOT KEY

It is important to make a rapid diagnosis during a patient's first psychotic break so that antipsychotic therapy can be started to reduce the frequency and severity of future episodes. Adequate, early treatment may have a beneficial effect on the long-term course of the illness.

II COURSE OF ILLNESS

A. **Risk factors** for schizophrenia include a family history of the illness, especially in first-degree relatives. Other associated factors include single marital status, lower socioeconomic class, living in an urban area, complications at birth, and a winter birth. Men and women are equally affected.

B. **Onset** is generally earlier in men (average onset, 22 years of age) than in women (average onset, 26 years of age). Onset may be sudden, but many patients experience a prodrome that may include poor hygiene, social isolation, odd behavior, odd beliefs, and lack of interest in school or work.

C. **Progression** of the disease is variable. After the first psychotic episode, some patients may remain free of future episodes and some may remain chronically psychotic. Most have a course marked by exacerbations and remissions. Most patients do not return to their premorbid level of functioning.

D. **Prognostic variables** can help predict the course of the illness.
   1. **Good prognostic variables** include female gender, late onset (after 45 years of age), acute onset, married status, good premorbid functioning, prominent mood symptoms, high intelligence, no family history of schizophrenia, family history of mood disorders, mainly positive symptoms, and good support systems.
   2. **Poor prognostic variables** include young age of onset, insidious onset, poor premorbid functioning, single marital status, family

history of schizophrenia, mainly negative symptoms, poor support systems, multiple relapses, and history of assaultiveness.

III DIAGNOSIS

A. **Criteria** for the diagnosis according to the DSM-IV include delusions, hallucinations, disorganized speech, disorganized behavior, and negative symptoms.
   1. Two or more of these symptoms must be present during a 1-month period. Only one symptom is required if a delusion is bizarre or if a hallucination is of two voices conversing or of a voice continuously commenting on the patient's behavior or thought.
   2. In addition, patients must experience marked social and occupational dysfunction for at least 6 months.
B. **Positive and negative symptoms** are terms that are used to categorize the symptoms of schizophrenia. **Positive symptoms** can be thought of as an **excess of normal functions** and **negative symptoms** as a **loss of normal functions.**
   1. **Positive symptoms** include delusions, hallucinations, and disorganized speech and behavior.
   2. **Negative symptoms** include **affective flattening,** or decreased emotional expression, **alogia,** or poverty of speech, and **avolition,** or decreased goal-directed behavior. Negative symptoms are responsible for much of the patient's interepisode dysfunction and are **difficult to treat.**
C. **Subtypes.** The subtypes of schizophrenia are easy to remember using the following mnemonic:

The subtypes of schizophrenia (**P**aranoid **C**athy **U**ndergoes **R**epeated **D**elusions)

Paranoid type
Catatonic type
Undifferentiated type
Residual type
Disorganized type

---

1. **Paranoid type** is characterized by prominent delusions, usually persecutory or grandiose, or auditory hallucinations. Symptoms commonly seen in disorganized or catatonic type (disorganized speech and behavior, flat affect) are generally absent. Age of onset is generally later, and the prognosis is better than for other subtypes.
2. **Catatonic type** involves psychomotor abnormalities that can include posturing, rigidity, stupor, mutism, or mannerisms.

   3. Undifferentiated type is a category for patients with active symptoms who do not meet the criteria for any of the other subtypes.
   4. Residual type is for patients who have had an acute episode of schizophrenia but who no longer have positive symptoms. They continue to have negative symptoms or marked functional impairment.
   5. Disorganized type is notable for disorganized speech, disorganized behavior, and flat affect. Patients with this type can show childlike or disinhibited behavior and have difficulty meeting their daily needs.
D. Differential diagnosis. Psychosis is defined as loss of contact with reality and can include symptoms such as delusions, hallucinations, disorganized speech or behavior, paranoid ideation, and ideas of reference. Before making the diagnosis of schizophrenia, other causes of psychosis must be ruled out. The differential diagnosis is very large and includes other psychiatric conditions that can manifest with psychosis, as well as medical, neurologic, and toxicologic conditions (see Chapter 9 II and III). The diagnosis is made using information about the onset and course of illness, medical history, family history, mental status, physical examination, and laboratory studies.

IV ETIOLOGY

A. The **stress-diathesis model** integrates biological, psychological, and social factors. The theory is that people who develop the illness have a genetic vulnerability to environmental stressors.
B. Structural brain changes have been found using computed tomography (CT) and magnetic resonance imaging (MRI) scans and postmortem studies. Some schizophrenic patients, especially those with predominantly negative symptoms, have enlarged ventricles and decreased volume and density in the limbic and frontal areas.
C. Neurochemical models have been developed for the pathogenesis of schizophrenia. The most widely accepted theory is the **dopamine theory,** which states that excess dopamine activity in the brain leads to the development of symptoms. Drugs that deplete dopamine or block dopamine receptors lead to a decrease in symptoms. Data also point to serotonin and norepinephrine dysfunction.
D. Genetic factors play a role in the development of schizophrenia. A child with one schizophrenic parent has about a 12% chance of developing the disorder. With two schizophrenic parents, the risk is about 40%. The risk, or concordance rate, in monozygotic (identical) twins is 40%–50%.
E. Psychosocial factors generally indicate that environmental

stress can lead to relapse. Studies have shown that the risk of relapse is greater for patients with families that have **high expressed emotion** (highly critical, hostile, or overinvolved).

HOT

Studies indicate that family dysfunction probably does **not** play a causative role in schizophrenia.

KEY

V APPROACH TO THE PATIENT

A. **Mental status examination** should be performed with particular attention paid to appearance (bizarre clothing, disheveled), behavior (mannerisms, posturing, relatedness to interviewer), affect (inappropriate, flat), thought process (illogical, tangential), thought content (delusions, hallucinations, paranoid ideation, ideas of reference, thought broadcasting), insight (degree of awareness of illness). (See Chapter 3.)

B. **Potential for suicide and violence** must be assessed in every patient. The patient must be questioned about suicidal ideation, intent or plan, command hallucinations (voices telling the patient to harm self or others), and violent thoughts. Past history of self-harm or violence should be obtained. If the patient seems to be dangerous to self or others, appropriate precautions must be taken (hospitalization, constant observation).

1. **History** of the symptoms is important, particularly onset and duration, and whether prodromal symptoms were present. Question whether there is a **family history** of schizophrenia or mood disorder. A **psychosocial history** should also be obtained including the patient's current level of functioning, premorbid level of functioning, history of substance use, and whether there is a support system (family, friends).

2. **Physical examination and laboratory studies** are important to rule out other illnesses. The physical examination should include a **neurologic examination**. A **urine drug screen** should be done to rule out recent substance use. Basic laboratory studies should be obtained including a **complete blood cell (CBC) count, electrolyte and glucose levels, liver function test, thyroid function tests,** and a **rapid plasmin reagin test (RPR). Human immunodeficiency virus (HIV) testing** should be obtained when indicated. A **head CT** may be warranted in a first episode of psychosis in a young person but is probably not necessary if the neurologic examination is normal and there is no history of head trauma. An **electroencephalogram (EEG)** should be considered if seizure disorder is suspected.

VI TREATMENT

A. Pharmacological therapy is fundamental in treating acute schizo-phrenic episodes and in preventing future episodes (see Chapter 11). The goals of acute treatment are to prevent harm, control ag-itated behavior, decrease symptoms, and improve functioning. Treatment with antipsychotic medications should be started within days, even if a definitive diagnosis cannot be made. The choice of medication is often made according to potential side ef-fects, including tardive dyskinesia. Anticholinergic medication may be added for prophylaxis against extrapyramidal symptoms (EPS). If the patient is agitated, benzodiazepines may be used. Once the acute episode has resolved, the patient should remain on the medication for at least 6 months to prevent relapse. After that, the dose can be very slowly reduced to the lowest dose needed to control symptoms and prevent relapse. Patients usu-ally need to be kept on antipsychotics indefinitely.

B. Psychosocial interventions should be used in the short-term and long-term treatment of schizophrenia. The goal of these inter-ventions is to decrease symptoms, prevent relapse, and help the patient obtain the highest level of functioning possible. Inter-ventions include supportive psychotherapy with the patient, working with the family to provide education about the illness and to reduce stress within the family, group therapy, cognitive and social skills training, and vocational training.

C. Noncompliance is a major cause of relapse. In a noncompliant patient, long-acting depot preparations of antipsychotics can be used (Haldol Decanoate injections every 4 weeks or Prolixin Decanoate injections every 2 weeks). In addition, the patient and family should be educated about the course of illness, the symptoms, the role of medication, and side effects.

VII COMORBIDITY

A. Almost 50% of patients with schizophrenia currently or previ-ously abused alcohol or illegal drugs. Substance abuse leads to worsening of psychotic symptoms and noncompliance with treatment. Patients with schizophrenia and substance abuse re-quire treatment of both conditions.

B. Depression occurs commonly in patients with schizophrenia. It often manifests as a **postpsychotic depression.**

HOT KEY The diagnosis of depression is often missed because the symp-toms may be confused with psychosis, negative symptoms, or medication side effects.

Because of the high risk of suicide, schizophrenic patients with depressive symptoms should be assessed for suicidal thoughts and treated with an antidepressant if necessary.

References

American Psychiatric Association: Practice guidelines for the treatment of patients with schizophrenia. *Am J Psychiatry* 154:1a–63a, 1997.

Lieberman JA: Pathophysiologic mechanisms in the pathogenesis and clinical course of schizophrenia. *J Clin Psychiatry* 60(suppl 12):9–12, 1999.

Wright IC, Rabe-Hesketh S, Woodruff PW, et al: Meta-analysis of regional brain volumes in schizophrenia. *Am J Psychiatry* 157:16–25, 2000.

11. Antipsychotic Medication

I INTRODUCTION

A. **Antipsychotic medications** are used to treat psychotic symptoms such as hallucinations, delusions, paranoia, disorganized speech, and disorganized behavior, as well as associated symptoms such as agitation and irritability.

B. Antipsychotic medications are commonly divided into **typical antipsychotics** and **atypical antipsychotics** according to their mechanisms of action and side effect profiles.

II MECHANISMS OF ACTION

A. The causes of psychosis are poorly understood. Much of what is currently known comes from research on schizophrenia.

   1. According to the **dopamine theory of schizophrenia** (see Chapter 10 IV C), excess in dopaminergic activity in the central nervous system plays a key role in the development of symptoms.

   2. Recently, data have also implicated dysregulation of **serotonin.**

B. The pharmacological treatment of psychotic symptoms is poorly understood but is thought to be based on the ways the medications affect one or both of these neurotransmitter systems.

   1. **Typical antipsychotics**

      a. These agents are thought to act on psychosis mainly by **central blockade of dopamine receptors** in the limbic and cortical areas.

      b. They also block dopamine receptors in the basal ganglia, which leads to their neurologic side effects, known as **extrapyramidal symptoms (EPS)** (see section III B 1).

      c. All typical antipsychotics are equally effective in treating symptoms, but their side effect profiles vary, according to how much anticholinergic, sedative, and hypotensive activity they have.

         (1) **High-potency** antipsychotics, such as haloperidol (Haldol), have **less anticholinergic activity** and have **more EPS.** They also have less sedating and hypotensive effects.

         (2) **Low-potency** antipsychotics, such as chlorpromazine (Thorazine), have **more anticholinergic activity** and **less EPS.** They have more sedating and hypotensive effects.

   2. Atypical antipsychotics
   a. These antipsychotic agents are newer and are thought to
      work by **blocking serotonin receptors** in addition to
      dopamine receptors.
   b. The atypical antipsychotics have very important advan-
      tages over the typical psychotics in that they cause **minimal
      EPS,** may have **less risk of tardive dyskinesia (TD),** and
      may be effective in treating negative symptoms (symptoms
      commonly seen in schizophrenia that include apathy, an-
      hedonia, affective flattening, and social isolation).
   c. Clozapine (Clozaril), the first atypical antipsychotic to be
      used clinically, is the only atypical antipsychotic shown to
      be effective in **treatment-refractory schizophrenia** and
      possibly to be effective in **treating TD.** The other atypical
      antipsychotics currently approved in the United States
      are **risperidone (Risperdal), olanzapine (Zyprexa),** and
      quetiapine (Seroquel).
3. Depot preparations are long-acting medications that can be
   given by injection at intervals from every 2 weeks to every 4
   weeks. Only haloperidol **(Haldol Decanoate)** and fluphenazine,
   (Prolixin Decanoate) are available in this long-acting form.
   These are very useful in treating patients who are noncompliant with oral medications.

III **SIDE EFFECTS.** Because antipsychotics affect a number
of neurotransmitter systems (dopaminergic, serotonergic,
adrenergic, cholinergic, histaminergic), they can have an array of side effects, ranging from those that are merely irritat-
ing to those that are life-threatening. They are categorized
here as non-neurologic side effects, neurologic side effects,
and side effects of unknown causes.

A. Non-neurologic side effects are numerous. Some are transient
   and may be managed with supportive measures or temporary
   dose reduction. Others require a change to another medication.
   The following is a list of the more common side effects.
   1. Sedation can be seen with any antipsychotic but is most com-
      mon with the high-potency typical antipsychotics, such as
      chlorpromazine (Thorazine) and thioridazine (Mellaril). It
      can also be seen with the atypical antipsychotics. This side ef-
      fect can be useful for calming an agitated patient early in
      treatment and for treating insomnia in a psychotic patient.
      This side effect is thought to be mediated through the action
      of histamine receptors.
   2. Postural hypotension is most severe with the low-potency
      medications and may be seen with atypical antipsychotics. It
      can be a problem for elderly patients. It can be treated by en-

couraging the patient to drink fluids and not to stand up
quickly. If severe, it may require dose reduction or a change
to a higher potency medication. This side effect is caused by
blockade of the α_1 receptor.

3. **Anticholinergic** side effects are more common with the low-
potency medications and include blurred vision, dry mouth,
urinary retention, and constipation. These side effects are often transient. If they persist, dose reduction or medication
change may be necessary.

4. **Hyperprolactinemia** can be a problem with all antipsychotics, except some of the atypical antipsychotics. It is due
to dopamine blockade in the hypothalamus where dopamine
normally acts to inhibit prolactin release. It can cause gyne-
comastia and galactorrhea in men and women, impotence in
men, and amenorrhea in women.

5. **Weight gain** is a problem with all antipsychotics and is a frequent cause of noncompliance with medication. The cause of
the weight gain is not known. Patients should be encouraged
to exercise and follow a diet.

6. **Agranulocytosis** is a serious and potentially fatal side effect
that is a major concern when prescribing the atypical antipsychotic clozapine. The incidence of agranulocytosis with clozapine is 1%–2% (versus 0.1% with typical antipsychotics). Patients on clozapine have to be cleared through a national
registry and weekly white blood cell counts must be obtained.

HOT

KEY

The presence of fever or signs of infection in patients taking
clozapine require urgent medical evaluation.

B. Neurologic side effects

1. **EPS** are likely the most common reason for noncompliance
with antipsychotics as they can be very disturbing and disabling to the patient. They are generally seen most often with
the high-potency antipsychotics, less with the low-potency
medications, and least with the atypical antipsychotics. Although the mechanism is not well understood, they are
thought to be due to dopamine blockade in the basal ganglia
causing a dopaminergic-cholinergic imbalance.

   a. **Acute dystonic reaction** presents as muscle spasms, usually
   in the eyes, tongue, jaw, or neck, and can be very frightening for the patient. Although it is rare, acute laryngospasm
   can lead to airway obstruction and is a medical emergency.
   Acute dystonia occurs within hours or days of starting a
   medication or increasing the dose. Young male African-

American patients are at highest risk. It can be treated acutely with benztropine (Cogentin), 2 mg intramuscularly, or diphenhydramine (Benadryl), 50 mg intramuscularly. Patients at higher risk can be treated prophylactically with benztropine (Cogentin), 1 to 2 mg orally twice a day.

b. Parkinsonism includes akinesia, rigidity, and tremor.

The symptoms of Parkinsonism are easy to remember—we have a patient named "ART" who has all three symptoms:

Akinesia
Rigidity
Tremor

Patients may complain of "shaking," feeling "stiff," or feeling "like a zombie." These symptoms usually develop several weeks after starting a medication. They can be confused with depressive symptoms or negative symptoms of schizophrenia. The elderly are at higher risk. Prophylaxis with anticholinergic medications, such as benztropine or diphenylhydramine, may be undertaken when initiating antipsychotic treatment.

c. Akathisia is motor restlessness that often manifests as pacing and fidgety leg movements while seated. It can be experienced by the patient as very distressing. It can occur after one dose of medication or after a dose is increased and can be confused with agitation due to psychosis. Treatment is with anticholinergic agents or β-blockers (e.g., propranolol). If it persists, a dose reduction or change to another antipsychotic may be required.

2. Tardive dyskinesia (TD) is a syndrome of abnormal involuntary movements that can involve the tongue and lips, hands, limbs, and trunk. It generally develops after months to years on antipsychotic medication and can range from mild movements to gross, disfiguring ones. All the typical antipsychotics can cause TD. The atypical antipsycotic clozapine does not seem to cause TD and may improve the symptoms in patients who have developed them while taking other antipsychotics. The other atypical antipsychotics are thought to have a lower risk of TD but long-term studies have yet to be done. The lowest antipsychotic doses needed to control symptoms should be used to reduce risk. TD is often untreatable.

C. Side effects of unknown cause include **neuroleptic malignant syndrome,** a potentially fatal side effect that can develop within

days to weeks of starting a neuroleptic (i.e., antipsychotic) drug
or increasing the dose. The symptoms are fever of at least 38°C,
rigidity and other neurologic signs, autonomic dysfunction (labile blood pressure, tachycardia, diaphoresis), and altered mental status. Laboratory studies can show leukocytosis and an elevated creatinine kinase level. The mortality rate is high.
Administration of antipsychotics should be stopped immediately. Treatment is mainly supportive (e.g., hydration) but can
also include administering dantrolene sodium or bromocriptine.

IV CHOOSING AN ANTIPSYCHOTIC (Tables 11-1 and 11-2).
The choice of an antipsychotic may be based on a number of
factors including a patient's age, medical problems, history of
response to a particular medication, and cost of the medication. In general, **low-potency antipsychotics** have more anti-

TABLE 11-1. Antipsychotics: Typical Therapeutic Doses			
Drug	**Chlorpromazine Equivalent (mg)**	**Relative Potency**	**Therapeutic Dose (mg/day)***
Chlorpromazine (Thorazine)	100	Low	150–2000
Triflupromazine (Vesprin)	30	Medium	20–150
Thioridazine (Mellaril)	100	Low	100–800
Mesoridazine (Serentil)	50	Medium	10–400
Perphenazine (Trilafon)	10	Medium	8–64
Trifluoperazine (Stelazine)	3–5	High	5–60
Fluphenazine (Prolixin)	3–5	High	5–60
Acetophenazine (Tindal)	15	Medium	20–100
Chlorprothixene (Taractan)	75	Low	100–600
Thiothixene (Navane)	3–5	High	5–60
Loxapine (Loxitane)	10–15	Medium	30–250
Haloperidol (Haldol)	2–5	High	2–100
Molindone (Moban)	5–10	Medium	10–225
Pimozide (Orap)	1–2	High	2–20
Clozapine (Clozaril)	100	Low	150–600
Risperidone (Risperdal)	0.6	High	4–16
Olanzapine (Zyprexa)	2–5	Low	5–20
Quetiapine (Seroquel)	70–100	Low	150–750

Modified from Kaplan HI, Sadock BJ: *Pocket Handbook of Clinical Psychiatry,*
2nd ed. Baltimore, Williams & Wilkins, 1996.
  *Extreme range.

TABLE 11-2. Antipsychotic Drug Interactions

Drug	Consequence
Tricyclic antidepressants	Increased concentration of both
Anticholinergics	Anticholinergic toxicity, decreased absorption of antipsychotics
Antacids	Decreased absorption of antipsychotics
Cimetidine	Decreased absorption of antipsychotics
Food	Decreased absorption of antipsychotics
Buspirone	Elevation of haloperidol levels
Barbiturates	Increased metabolism of antipsychotics, excessive sedation
Phenytoin	Decreased phenytoin metabolism
Guanethidine	Reduced hypotensive effect
Clonidine	Reduced hypotensive effect
α-Methyldopa	Reduced hypotensive effect
Levodopa	Decreased effects of both
Succinylcholine	Prolonged muscle paralysis
Monoamine oxidase inhibitors	Hypotension
Halothane	Hypotension
Alcohol	Potentiation of CNS depression
Cigarettes	Decreased plasma levels of antipsychotics
Epinephrine	Hypotension
Propranolol	Increased plasma concentration of both
Warfarin	Decreased plasma concentrations of warfarin

From Kaplan HI, Sadock BJ: *Pocket Handbook of Clinical Psychiatry,* 2nd ed. Baltimore, Williams & Wilkins, 1996.
CNS = central nervous system.

cholinergic and sedating side effects and fewer EPS. **High-potency antipsychotics** have more risk of EPS but are less sedating and less anticholinergic. **Atypicals** cause very few EPS and there is thought to be little or no risk of TD. However, atypical antipsychotics are very costly. In addition, clozapine requires compliance with weekly white blood cell counts.

 INFORMED CONSENT. Informed consent is important when beginning any antipsychotic regimen. Informed consent consists of a patient's voluntary consent to treatment after being adequately educated about the proposed treatment. It is important to explain the risks and benefits of

treatment with a medication, including the risk of TD. Informed consent cannot occur if the patient does not have the
ability for rational decision making, and this can be difficult
with an acutely psychotic patient. When faced with the difficult situation of an acutely psychotic patient with impaired
capacity for judgment, it may be necessary to get a court order to treat despite the patient's objection.

References

American Psychiatric Association: Practice guideline for the treatment of patients with
    schizophrenia. *Am J Psychiatry* 154:1a–63a, 1997.
De Quardo JR: Pharmacologic treatment of first-episode schizophrenia: Early inter-
    vention is key to outcome. *J Clin Psychiatry* 59(suppl 19):9–17, 1998.
Fleischhacker WW: Clozapine: A comparison with other novel antipsychotics. *J Clin
    Psychiatry* 60(suppl 12):30–34, 1999.
The Expert Consensus Guideline Series: Treatment of schizophrenia 1999. *J Clin Psy-
    chiatry* 60(suppl 11):1–80, 1999.

PART IV

Substance Abuse

12. Alcohol Abuse and Dependence

I INTRODUCTION

A. Alcohol is the most commonly used substance of abuse.

B. Its abuse is associated with numerous physical and psychological manifestations that the clinician may face in the emergency department, or inpatient and outpatient settings.

C. Alcohol abuse and dependence are extremely common, with a lifetime prevalence approaching 15%. About one hundred thousand Americans die each year from complications of alcohol use.

D. Despite this, alcohol abuse and dependence are often underdiagnosed and undertreated.

HOT
KEY

Almost 25% of Americans say that drinking has been a source of trouble in their families.

II CLINICAL MANIFESTATIONS OF SUBSTANCE ABUSE AND DEPENDENCE.

Although alcohol abuse is extremely common, the majority of alcohol users have not developed physical dependence and do not regularly overindulge in alcohol. The **DSM-IV** outlines criteria for what constitutes abuse and dependence for alcohol, opiates, cocaine, and other substances.

A. Substance abuse

1. **General definition.** Substance abuse is a maladaptive pattern of substance use, leading to clinically significant impairment or distress.

2. **The DSM-IV criteria** for substance abuse include **lack of**

control of use, and the consequences of use lead to **distress or impairment in cognitive, social, or occupational spheres.** They differ from the criteria for dependence in that tolerance and withdrawal are not present. If **one or more of the following** has been present over the past year, the patient is a substance abuser:

   a. Recurrent substance use resulting in a failure to **fulfill major role obligations** at work, school, or home
   b. Recurrent substance use in situations in which it is **physically hazardous**
   c. Recurrent substance-related **legal problems**
   d. Continued substance use despite having **persistent or recurrent social or interpersonal problems** caused or exacerbated by the effects of the substance

B. Substance dependence
   1. General definition. Substance dependence leads to **distress and impairment** (like substance abuse though perhaps to a greater degree), and also includes **signs of physical dependence, tolerance, and withdrawal symptoms.**
   2. DSM-IV criteria for substance dependence (three or more of the following must be present over a 12-month period):
      a. Tolerance
         (1) A **need for markedly increased amounts** of the substance to achieve intoxication
         (2) Markedly diminished effect with continued use of the same amount of the substance
      b. Withdrawal
         (1) Characteristic **withdrawal syndrome** for the substance
         (2) Same or closely related **substance is taken to relieve or avoid withdrawal symptoms**
      c. Lack of control in use patterns (one or more of the following must be present):
         (1) Substance is taken in **larger amounts or over a longer period** than was intended.
         (2) There are **persistent desires or unsuccessful efforts to cut down** or control substance use.
      d. Problematic consequences (one of the following must be present):
         (1) A great deal of time is spent in activities necessary to obtain the substance, use the substance, or recover from its effects.
         (2) Important social, occupational, or recreational **activities are given up or reduced** because of substance use.
         (3) The substance use is **continued despite awareness** that a persistent or recurrent physical or psychologi-

cal problem is present that is likely to have been caused or exacerbated by the substance.

III CLINICAL MANIFESTATIONS OF ALCOHOL INTOXICATION AND WITHDRAWAL

A. Alcohol intoxication
   1. Intoxication is an important red flag to detect in an alcohol user.

Intoxication symptoms typically progress in the following order, which can be easily remembered using the mnemonic "Ed Sips Drinks Most Afternoons."

Euphoria
Slurred speech
Disinhibition
Mood lability
Ataxia

HOT
KEY

Severe intoxication can lead to respiratory depression, coma, and death.

   2. DSM-IV criteria for intoxication are based on measuring blood alcohol levels (BALs).
   a. Levels are described in mg% (or mg/100 ml blood or mg/dl), with anything above 0.08%–0.15% (80–150 mg/100 ml) being "legally intoxicated" in most states (too drunk to drive).
   b. Serious alcohol intoxication with blackouts occurs in the nontolerant individual at BALs above 300 mg/dl (0.3%).
   c. Levels above 400 mg/dl (0.4%) can cause coma and death.
   d. In someone who has become dependent on alcohol, the degree of tolerance that develops may allow them to be awake and talking at BALs that would be lethal to nontolerant individuals (e.g., > 0.4%).

B. Alcohol withdrawal
   1. Initial symptoms of alcohol withdrawal emerge as the BAL begins to decline, usually within a few hours of the last drink.
   2. Delirium tremens (DTs) is an extreme form of alcohol withdrawal that occurs in up to 5% of patients withdrawing

from alcohol. Its onset is usually within 72 hours after cessation of drinking but can occur up to 1 week later.

Order of progression of alcohol withdrawal symptoms: "Tom's Thinking About Stopping Drinking Today."

Tremulousness—within hours.
Temperature, pulse, and blood pressure increase—within hours
Anxiety, psychomotor **A**gitation, and **A**uditory and, more often, visual hallucinations—12–24 hours after the last drink
Seizures—48–72 hours after drinking stops
Delirium **T**remens (DTs)

HOT KEY

The mortality rate of patients with DTs is 20%; thus, all patients with DTs should be hospitalized.

---

    a. Symptoms of DTs include **waxing and waning consciousness (delirium), agitation,** and autonomic hyperactivity. Visual and auditory **hallucinations** are common during DTs.
    b. DTs must be treated aggressively with benzodiazepines for withdrawal symptoms and supportive care to manage autonomic instability.
    c. With hospitalization and proper care, symptoms usually resolve within 1–5 days.

HOT KEY

Delirium occurring in the context of alcohol withdrawal may also signal concurrent medical illness such as hepatic failure, pancreatitis, infection, or fall-related injury including fracture or subdural hematoma.

IV APPROACH TO THE PATIENT

A. Assessment of substance use patterns. All patients should be screened for alcohol use, given the high prevalence of alcohol abuse and the proven effectiveness of intervention. Numerous screening tools have been developed.
    1. CAGE questions. One of the simplest screening tools is the **CAGE** that asks the following four questions:

Questions to screen for alcohol abuse ("CAGE")

Have you ever:
tried to **C**ut down on your drinking?
been **A**nnoyed by others' comments about your drinking?
felt **G**uilty about drinking?
had an **E**ye-opener (a drink) first thing in the morning to
   calm your nerves or counteract a hangover?

2. **Other questions** to ask include:
   a. How many drinks do you have in an average week?
   b. On a typical day, how many drinks do you have?
   c. What is the maximum number of drinks you have had on
      any occasion in the past month?

HOT KEY

The quantity of drinks is not as important as the **effect that alcohol has on the person's life,** such as charges of driving while intoxicated (DWI) or driving under the influence of alcohol (DUI), missing days of work, and frequent arguments with family members.

B. **Assessment of psychiatric comorbidity**
   1. Always evaluate for the presence of other comorbid conditions such as **depression and anxiety.**
   2. In diagnosing comorbid conditions, it is important to see if mood or psychotic symptoms, for instance, are experienced only in the context of substance abuse (either while intoxicated or in withdrawal) or while the patient was sober. That is, if the psychiatric symptoms are **alcohol induced,** the diagnosis should be clearly indicated as such (e.g., alcohol induced mood disorder, alcohol-induced anxiety disorder). The most important treatment consideration in this regard is that maintaining sobriety can often cure the associated symptoms.
C. **Assessment of medical comorbidity**
   1. A **physical examination with laboratory testing** should be part of your assessment of every alcohol user.
   2. There are many **medical complications from chronic alcohol abuse.** Some of the most common are:
      a. Gastrointestinal disorders (e.g., gastritis, hepatitis, cirrhosis, esophageal varices, pancreatitis)
      b. Neurologic disorders (e.g., peripheral neuropathy, Wernicke's encephalopathy, dementia)
      c. Cardiovascular disorders (e.g., hypertension, cardiomyopathy)

   d. Hematologic disorders (e.g., anemia, thrombocytopenia)
   e. Endocrine and metabolic disorders (e.g., hypoglycemia, ketoacidosis, hypokalemia, hyponatremia)
   f. Trauma (e.g., automobile accidents, falls, domestic violence)

V TREATMENT

A. Alcoholic intoxication
   1. A BAL should be obtained.
   2. In a seriously intoxicated patient, gastric lavage with 50 g of 50% glucose should be administered to prevent hypoglycemia, ICU monitoring should be maintained, and thiamine, 100 mg, should be administered intramuscularly to prevent Wernicke's encephalopathy.
   3. The patient should also be monitored for signs and symptoms of alcohol withdrawal and treated appropriately.

HOT KEY   Symptoms of withdrawal begin when alcohol level falls, meaning that a patient may be in alcohol withdrawal while still intoxicated.

B. Alcohol withdrawal
   1. Medication. The psychopharmacology of alcohol dependence is complex and involves multiple neurotransmitters.
      a. Treatment of withdrawal requires giving tapering doses of a medication with cross-tolerance to alcohol, which includes **benzodiazepines or barbiturates.**
      b. Other drugs, including anticonvulsants, β-blockers, and α-adrenergic agonists, have also been used for alcohol detoxification; however, they do not appear to be as effective as the benzodiazepines and may entail higher risks.

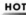

HOT KEY   In patients over 60 years of age and those with severe chronic obstructive pulmonary disease, use lower doses of benzodiazepines and monitor closely for excess sedation or respiratory distress or failure.

---

      c. Usually, a benzodiazepine such as chlordiazepoxide (Librium) is used.
         (1) The dosing regimen starts with 50 mg orally every 6 hours for four doses, followed by a reduction to 25 mg orally every 6 hours for four doses, then to 10 mg orally every 6 hours, and then discontinuation. This regimen will be sufficient for the majority of patients.

      (2) Caution should be used in treating patients with liver disease because they will be slower to metabolize chlordiazepoxide (Librium). An alternative would be lorazepam (Ativan) because it is not metabolized by the liver. A starting dose of 1–2 mg lorazepam orally every 6 hours, tapering by 0.5 mg every 24 hours, should be sufficient.

  2. Nutritional support. All patients requiring detoxification should receive nutritional support including high caloric intake as well as high doses of vitamins:

    a. Thiamine, 100 mg orally daily
    b. Folic acid, 1 mg orally daily
    c. Multivitamins, including all of the B vitamins

C. Treatment of comorbid illnesses is also important. There are some alcohol-dependent patients in recovery who may require treatment with benzodiazepines for comorbid panic or other anxiety disorders. This should be done with caution because there is potential for abuse of the benzodiazepines. The decision to treat should be based on persistent anxiety symptoms, despite a reasonable period of sobriety occurring prior to the period of alcohol abuse.

D. Rehabilitation. Most patients requiring detoxification will require further time to acclimate to sobriety. Formally, this treatment phase is called "rehabilitation" because patients learn how to live without drinking.

  1. Program types include short-term and long-term inpatient alcohol rehabilitation programs, therapeutic communities (TCs), and outpatient programs.

  2. Self-help groups such as Alcoholics Anonymous and Smart Recovery are often used as adjuncts to rehabilitation programs.

  3. Selection of a program is a decision that requires consideration of employment status, insurance, and family commitments and is often done with the help of an alcohol counselor or social worker.

E. Medications for maintaining sobriety. Though there are no medications that are effective in resolving alcohol dependence, some benefit may be gained through supplemental medications during recovery.

  1. Disulfiram (Antabuse) interferes with the metabolism of acetaldehyde, which accumulates in the blood after alcohol use. It serves as an aversive therapy because if alcohol is used while on the medication, the patient will experience severe unpleasant symptoms (e.g., flushing, vasodilation, headache, tachycardia, diaphoresis, hyperventilation, nausea, vomiting) for 1–3 hours.

    a. The dosing regimen for disulfiram is as follows: After the patient is alcohol-free for 4–5 days, therapy should be initiated with a dosage of 500 mg orally daily for 1–3 weeks; the maintenance dosage is 250–500 mg daily for as long as the patient requires this extra assurance in maintaining sobriety (often several months or a couple of years). The effects of disulfiram may last for 3–7 days after the last dose.

  b. Side effects include optic neuritis, peripheral neuropathy, rash, and hepatitis (rare). Psychotic reactions, which are also rare, are associated with a high dosage or combined drug toxicity (particularly with metronidazole or isoniazid).

  c. Contraindications include acute hepatitis, significant cardiac disease, pregnancy, severe chronic lung disease, suicidal ideation, rubber allergy, occupational exposure to solvents or alcohol, and the concurrent use of metronidazole or isoniazid.

 2. Naltrexone decreases alcohol craving, probably by blocking the release of endogenous opioids associated with alcohol use.

  a. Therapy should be initiated as soon as withdrawal symptoms have resolved (usually 3 to 5 days).

  b. An initial dose of 25 mg daily can be titrated to 50 mg daily.

  c. Naltrexone aids in achieving abstinence by reducing alcohol craving. Naltrexone alone, however, has not been proven to be an effective treatment for most patients, so it must be combined with AA meetings and other forms of treatment to maintain sobriety.

  d. Because naltrexone is an opioid antagonist, severe opioid withdrawal syndromes can be precipitated by the administration of naltrexone in opioid-dependent persons. **Screen for concomitant opioid abuse before prescribing.**

References

Hall W, Zador D: The alcohol withdrawal syndrome. *Lancet* 349(9069):1897–1900, 1997.

O'Connor PG, Schottenfeld RS: Patients with alcohol problems. *N Engl J Med* 338(9):592–602, 1998.

Swift RM: Drug therapy for alcohol dependence. *N Engl J Med* 340(19):1482–1490, 1999.

Tinsley JA, Finlayson RE, Morse RM: Developments in the treatment of alcoholism. *Mayo Clinic Proc* 73(9):857–863, 1998.

13. Opioid Abuse and Dependence

I INTRODUCTION

A. Opioids include all of the following:
   1. Naturally occurring substances such as opium, morphine, and codeine.
   2. Semi-synthetic substances such as heroin, hydromorphone (Dilaudid), and oxycodone (Percodan).
   3. Synthetic substances including propoxyphene (Darvon), meperidine (Demerol), and methadone (Dolophine).
B. All of these drugs **can produce tolerance** and **dependence** and **have abuse potential** secondary to their reinforcing effects.

II CLINICAL MANIFESTATIONS OF OPIOID ABUSE AND DEPENDENCE

A. Because opiates are obtained either by illegal activity or by tricking a physician into prescribing them, it is often more readily apparent that an abuse or dependence problem exists than with alcohol.
B. The **DSM-IV criteria** for abuse and dependence of opioid substances follows the same outline as discussed in Chapter 12 II.

III CAUSES OF OPIOID DEPENDENCE.
Opioids bind to several receptors in the brain, with μ and δ receptors seemingly responsible for the reinforcing effects of the drugs. Stimulation of these receptors produces **euphoria and analgesia** as well as **central nervous system suppression.**

IV CLINICAL MANIFESTATIONS OF OPIOID INTOXICATION AND WITHDRAWAL

A. **Intoxication**
   1. Patients experience an initial rush upon intravenous use of heroin that has been described as orgasmic.
   2. All opioids cause:
      a. Changes in mood: often a sense of tranquility or decreased anxiety
      b. Sedation
      c. Decreased respiratory drive

    d. Constipation
    e. Bradycardia
    f. Hypothermia
    g. Pinpoint pupils unresponsive to light with the exception
       of meperidine (Demerol)

HOT KEY Ingestion of meperidine may produce dilated pupils secondary to anticholinergic effects.

The most important clinical manifestations of opioid overdose can be easily remembered using the mnemonic "DOPE."

Decreased respiratory drive
Obtundation
Pinpoint pupils
Euphoria

HOT KEY Opioid overdose is a medical emergency because it can lead to coma and death.

B. Withdrawal
    1. As with all drugs, **withdrawal produces the opposite effects of intoxication.** A **flu-like syndrome** ensues, involving:
      —Piloerection (going "cold turkey")
      —Rhinorrhea
      —Diarrhea
      —Vomiting
      —Achiness
      —Muscle cramps
      —Yawning
      —Dilated pupils
    2. Withdrawal symptoms emerge **8–12 hours after the last dose** of heroin **peaking within 48–72 hours** and resolving over 7–10 days.

HOT KEY Although withdrawal from opioids is very uncomfortable and the patient can appear to be in a lot of distress, uncomplicated opioid withdrawal is not life-threatening.

V APPROACH TO THE PATIENT

A. **Assessment of substance use pattern.** Be sure to evaluate patients for comorbid use of other substances (e.g., alcohol, cocaine, benzodiazepines).

B. **Evaluation of medical complications.** Intravenous heroin users should be evaluated for medical complications such as **cellulitis, phlebitis, abscesses, endocarditis, HIV, and hepatitis B and C.**

C. **Evaluation for detoxification programs.** If the patient is in distress about his drug use, wants to stop, and has no medical contraindications, a detox program should be offered.

D. **Assessment of psychiatric comorbidity.** Always evaluate for the presence of other psychiatric symptoms, such as mood or anxiety disorders. Be sure to differentiate as fully as possible those that are experienced only in the context of substance abuse (Chapter 12 IV B).

HOT

KEY
Heroin-related emergency department visits more than doubled from 1990 (33,900) to 1996 (70,500).

VI TREATMENT

A. **Treatment of opioid intoxication.** Opioid overdose is a medical emergency because of respiratory depression and possible obtundation. Management is as follows:
  1. Intensive care unit (ICU) monitoring is usually necessary.
  2. Treatment with **naloxone (Narcan)** 0.4–2.0 mg intravenously (IV) should be given every 2–3 minutes until respirations are stable.
  3. If the respiratory depression is not reversed after 10 mg of naloxone, other causes should be considered (e.g., overdose of benzodiazepines or alcohol).

HOT

KEY
The half-life of naloxone is much shorter than that of most opioids (approximately 1 hour), so observe closely for the reemergence of symptoms (respiratory depression and coma) and retreat with naloxone, if necessary.

---

  4. The patient should be monitored for withdrawal symptoms.
B. **Opioid detoxification**
  1. **Outpatient detoxification using clonidine.** Opioid users may undergo outpatient detoxification using clonidine (Catapres), an α_1-receptor agonist that treats most of the symptoms of

withdrawal by dampening adrenergic output. However, the patient should have a family member or friend dispense the medication and monitor the patient for any problems during the detoxification. The regimen involves prescribing clonidine 0.1 mg orally every 4–6 hours the first day and then increasing to 0.2 mg orally every 4–6 hours, not to exceed 1.2 mg per day over the next 2 days. The medication should then be tapered by 0.2 mg per day. Blood pressure should be monitored, and the medication should not be given if the blood pressure is less than 90/60. In addition, a benzodiazepine taper should be given to treat muscle cramps [e.g., **lorazepam (Ativan)** 1–2 mg orally every 6 hours for the first 3 days, and then tapered]. Supplemental medications can be used to treat other physical symptoms not fully covered by clonidine such as **prochlorperazine (Compazine)** suppositories (25 mg twice a day) to treat nausea and vomiting, **ibuprofen** (400–800 mg orally every 6 hours) to treat muscle aches, and **trazodone** (50 mg orally just before bedtime) to treat insomnia.

2. **Inpatient detoxification with methadone.** Patients who are using five or more bags of heroin, who are homeless, or who have medical complications may require inpatient detoxification with methadone. Methadone is primarily a μ opioid receptor agonist with some activity at the κ and δ receptors. This agonist activity blocks the symptoms associated with opioid withdrawal. Methadone has analgesic effects but does not cause the same euphoria as heroin because of its long half-life (approximately 24 hours). It is a schedule II drug, only allowed to be prescribed in hospitals, in prisons, or through designated clinics called methadone maintenance treatment programs (see VII B 1). Detoxification with methadone can begin with between 20 and 40 mg of methadone. When possible, the dose should be tapered by no more than approximately 20% per day. The dose can be given once a day or in divided doses up to four times daily. **Clonidine** can be used to supplement a methadone taper with a dose of 0.1–0.2 mg orally every 4–6 hours but should not be given if the blood pressure is below 90/60 mm Hg. Once the detoxification regimen is complete, a patient may still experience cravings and anxiety as well as other symptoms for up to several weeks. The patient should be counseled about this prior to beginning the detoxification, and preparation for further treatment should be started as soon as possible.

3. **Other possibilities for detoxification** include rapid detoxification—a naltrexone-precipitated withdrawal done under anesthesia. At this time, the risks of general anesthesia do not clearly outweigh the benefits of a rapid detoxification and further study of this technique is needed.

HOT KEY

The treatment of choice for pregnant heroin-addicted women is methadone maintenance at the lowest dose possible.

VII FOLLOW-UP AND REFERRAL

A. **Rehabilitation programs and support groups.** Most patients requiring detoxification will require further rehabilitation in order to keep from abusing opioids again.

1. Rehabilitation programs include **short-term and long-term inpatient rehabilitation programs, therapeutic communities,** and **outpatient programs.**

2. Selection of a program is a decision that requires consideration of employment status, insurance, and family commitments and is often done with the help of an alcohol counselor or social worker.

3. Support groups such as **Narcotics Anonymous** are often used as adjuncts to rehabilitation programs.

B. **Maintenance therapy**

1. **Methadone maintenance therapy.** Another treatment for patients who have been unsuccessful in their attempts to stop using heroin or other opioids is methadone maintenance therapy.

   a. There are approximately 600,000 heroin addicts in the United States and approximately 100,000 on methadone maintenance.

   b. Methadone is initiated at doses between 20 and 40 mg per day and then increased.

   c. The maintenance dose is set at the point at which cravings are eliminated and there is no longer illicit use of opioids. Average maintenance doses range from 30 to 100 mg.

2. There are other drugs being used for maintenance therapy that have the advantage of being dosed less frequently than methadone.

   a. L-Alpha-acetylmethadol, or **LAAM,** can be dosed three times per week because of the long half-lives of its active metabolites. Although it received FDA approval in 1993, it is still not widely available.

   b. Buprenorphine is a partial agonist at the μ receptor and is currently under investigation for maintenance therapy.

3. **Naltrexone for opioid dependence.** Naltrexone, a μ receptor antagonist, has been used in the treatment of opioid dependence.

   a. By binding competitively with the μ receptor, naltrexone blocks the euphoric effects of opioids.

  b. Because naltrexone is an opioid antagonist, severe opioid withdrawal syndromes can be precipitated by the administration of naltrexone in opioid-dependent persons.

  c. The clinician should be certain that the patient is opioid-free for at least 7 days before beginning treatment with naltrexone to prevent precipitation of withdrawal.

  d. Patients taking naltrexone should be cautioned that the effects of opioid-containing medicines, such as cough and cold preparations, antidiarrheal preparations, and opioid analgesics, will be diminished.

  e. In an emergency situation in which opioid analgesia must be administered to a patient receiving naltrexone, the amount of opioid required will be greater than usual, and the resulting respiratory depression may be deeper and more prolonged. Therefore, caution must be exercised.

References

Effective medical treatment of opiate addiction. National Consensus Development Panel on Effective Medical Treatment of Opiate Addiction. *JAMA* 280(22): 1936–1943, 1998.

O'Connor PG, Kosten TR: Rapid and ultrarapid opioid detoxification techniques. *JAMA* 279(3):229–234, 1998.

Sporer KA. Acute heroin overdose. *Ann Intern Med* 130:584–590, 1999.

Ward J, Hall W, Mattick RP: Role of maintenance treatment in opioid dependence. *Lancet* 353:221–226, 1999.

14. Other Drugs of Abuse

I INTRODUCTION

A. Chapters 12 and 13 discuss use of alcohol and opioid substances. Use of **other illicit drugs,** such as **psychostimulants, sedative-hypnotics, hallucinogens, marijuana, phencyclidine (PCP),** and **inhalants,** is also common.

B. Each of these drugs produces a different picture of intoxication and withdrawal.

C. Psychiatric symptoms often result from use of these drugs.

HOT

KEY
Approximately 13 million people (or 6% of the population) 12 years of age and over currently use illicit drugs.

II CLINICAL MANIFESTATIONS OF DRUG ABUSE

A. Psychostimulants. This class of drugs includes **cocaine, crack, and amphetamines.** Use of **caffeine** can produce similar symptoms but to a much milder degree.

 1. Intoxication symptoms of psychostimulants include:
  a. Euphoria
  b. Motor restlessness
  c. Decreased appetite and evidence of weight loss
  d. Signs of autonomic stimulation: hypertension, tachycardia

 2. Complications of intoxication. Taken in high doses, psychostimulants can lead to **psychosis** (paranoia and hallucinations), autonomic instability with **cardiac arrhythmias, hyperthermia, seizures, and coma. Stroke** and **myocardial infarction** can also occur due to extreme cocaine intoxication.

 3. Withdrawal symptoms from the psychostimulants can best be characterized as the **opposite of autonomic stimulation:**
  a. Fatigue or sleepiness
  b. Increased appetite
  c. Depressed mood, sometimes with suicidal ideation
  d. Psychomotor agitation

B. Sedative-hypnotics. This class of drugs includes **benzodiazepines, barbiturates** (e.g., phenobarbital), **glutethimide** (Doriden), and meprobamate (Equanil, Miltown). **Symptoms related to this class of drugs are similar to those produced by alcohol.**

1. **Intoxication symptoms—at low doses**
    a. Sedation
    b. Ataxia
    c. Slurred speech
    d. Nystagmus
2. **At high doses,** the symptoms can progress to:
    a. Decreased respiratory rate
    b. Confusion
    c. Decreased level of consciousness or even coma

HOT

KEY

Benzodiazepine overdose alone is rarely fatal. When combined with alcohol, however, fatal respiratory depression can occur.

---

3. **Withdrawal symptoms**
    a. Hypertension
    b. Tachycardia
    c. Tremulousness
    d. Nausea
    e. Vomiting
    f. Headache
    g. Anxiety
4. The withdrawal syndrome from sedative-hypnotics, like that of alcohol withdrawal, **may progress to seizures or delirium in 24–72 hours after last use.**
C. **Hallucinogens.** This class of drugs includes lysergic acid diethylamide **(LSD),** psilocybin **(mushrooms),** dimethoxymethylamphetamine **(STP or DOM),** mescaline **(peyote),** and methylenedioxymethamphetamine **(MDMA or XTC "ecstasy").**
    1. **Intoxication symptoms** include:
        a. Dilated pupils
        b. Tachycardia
        c. Hypertension
        d. Labile affect
        e. Alternating periods of hallucinations and lucidity
        f. Perceptual distortions including synesthesia (e.g., sound might be perceived as color)
    2. The effects may persist over several days.
        a. A **"bad trip"** may result, in which a patient can become psychotic or severely panicky.
        b. "Flashbacks" are a result of chronic LSD use and involve the reexperiencing of the hallucinatory experience.
    3. Withdrawal symptoms. **No significant withdrawal symptoms are seen with the hallucinogens.**

D. PCP and **ketamine ("Special K," a PCP analogue).** Although these drugs can cause hallucinations, they differ from the hallucinogens in that they can cause severe agitation and are lethal in very high doses.

1. **Intoxication symptoms**—at low doses
   a. Altered sense of self, depersonalization
   b. Ataxia
   c. Dysarthria
   d. Confusion
   e. Decreased sensitivity to pain
2. **At increasing doses,** intoxication with PCP or ketamine can lead to severe agitation, hallucinations, coma, and death.

HOT KEY

Unlike those of other drugs of abuse, symptoms of PCP intoxication can linger for weeks.

3. Withdrawal symptoms. **There is no significant withdrawal or tolerance that develops with these drugs.**

E. Marijuana and hashish

1. **Definition.** Marijuana and hashish, its more potent counterpart, have as their active metabolite tetrahydrocannabinol. Most commonly, these drugs are smoked or eaten. They do not cause physical dependence or significant tolerance.
2. **Intoxication symptoms** include:
   a. Euphoria or feeling of well-being
   b. Altered perceptions
   c. Incoordination
   d. Increased appetite ("the munchies")
   e. Tachycardia
   f. Injected conjunctivae
   g. Anxiety
   h. Paranoia

HOT KEY

Reality testing is intact with cannabis intoxication. If delirium is present, diagnosis of substance-induced psychotic disorder should be considered.

3. Withdrawal symptoms. **There are no significant withdrawal symptoms associated with marijuana or hashish.**

F. Inhalants. This class of drugs includes **gasoline products, some aerosols, glue, paint thinners, and nail polish remover.**

1. **Intoxication symptoms** include:
   a. Altered states ranging from euphoria to clouding of consciousness to psychosis
   b. Dizziness
   c. Nausea and vomiting
   d. Chest pain, arrhythmias
   e. Breath odor in some patients
2. **Withdrawal symptoms** include:
   a. Headache
   b. Nausea

III APPROACH TO THE PATIENT

A. **In general, intoxication can lead to very unpredictable and even violent behavior.**
   1. Initial assessment should include **vital signs** and evaluation for **physical trauma.**
   2. "Downers" tend to produce less agitation but greater confusion.
   3. **Cocaine users, especially chronic users, can be quite paranoid** and may develop auditory hallucinations with commands to hurt themselves or others.
   4. **PCP intoxication tends to lead to the greatest agitation.** When coupled with the grandiosity and decreased sensitivity to pain that usually accompany it, acts of violence and self-injury are common consequences.
B. **Physician strategies**
   1. First and foremost, the physician should be aware of the environment and her own safety.
   2. A calm, straightforward manner should be used, and back-up support from other staff should always be available.
   3. Any treatment should be explained to the patient to minimize paranoia and provide reality testing.
   4. Patients should be monitored for safety and not left alone.
   5. Attention to the patient's medical stability is critical.

IV TREATMENT

A. Treatment for **intoxication** with **stimulants, hallucinogens, marijuana, PCP,** or **inhalants** is as follows.
   1. Patients should be managed in a quiet room with diminished stimuli.
   2. **If a seizure has occurred, or if arrhythmia, hyperthermia, or significant hyper- or hypotension is present, the patient should be moved to an intensive care unit for medical monitoring.**
   3. If patients present with anticholinergic manifestations, treatment with **physostigmine** should be considered.
   4. For acute agitation, benzodiazepines such as **lorazepam**

(Ativan) 1–2 mg intramuscularly or intravenously every 1–2 hours should be administered until the patient is calm.

5. If the patient exhibits paranoia, neuroleptic medication can be used, such as haloperidol (Haldol) 5 mg given orally or intramuscularly every 1–2 hours in conjunction with benzodiazepines, until patient is calm.

6. Vital signs should continue to be monitored closely, and psychiatric symptoms reassessed periodically.

7. If symptoms persist beyond 24 hours, patients may need hospitalization for further observation.

HOT KEY Very high doses of cocaine can cause seizures, hyperthermia, tachycardia, and arrhythmias that need to be managed in an intensive care setting.

B. Treatment of **intoxication with sedative-hypnotics** is as follows:
1. If recent ingestion has taken place, **activated charcoal** and **gastric lavage** may be helpful.
2. The patient should be **hospitalized** with **monitoring of vital signs,** as overdose with many of these drugs can be fatal.
3. As the intoxication clears, the physician should **continue to evaluate for symptoms of withdrawal that could also be fatal** (seizures, autonomic instability) and **begin a detoxification regimen** if the patient appears to have become dependent on the substance.

C. **Detoxification treatment** for withdrawal from sedative-hypnotics is as follows:
1. Patients should be **treated with the specific substance of abuse in a tapering dose** if possible.
2. As a general rule, on the first day of detoxification, patients should be given enough medication to suppress withdrawal with some mild sedation.
3. Dosing should occur in regular intervals based on the half-life of the medication, and total dose should be decreased by no more than 20% per day.
4. Drugs with longer half-lives may require a slower taper.
5. Benzodiazepines and barbiturates have cross-tolerance and may be substituted for each other. (See Chapter 12 V B 1 c for an example of a benzodiazepine detoxification regimen.)

V FOLLOW-UP AND REFERRAL

A. Discharge from hospital
1. Once a patient is no longer intoxicated or in withdrawal, discharge from the hospital becomes possible. However, if significant comorbid psychiatric symptoms are present (such as

depressed mood, suicidal ideation, or paranoia), psychiatric treatment in an inpatient setting may be necessary. Ideally, continued substance abuse treatment would also be incorporated (e.g., in a "dual-diagnosis clinical unit").

2. Patients who no longer need hospitalization but fulfill criteria for substance abuse or dependence should be offered further treatment. Options are similar to those for rehabilitation of opioid abuse (see Chapter 13 VII A).

B. **Medications and treatment of underlying psychiatric symptoms.** Treatment of any underlying anxiety or mood symptoms **should ideally be undertaken after the patient has been substance-free for at least a month** to allow the influence of substances to be distinguished from psychiatric symptoms.

References

Boghdadi MS, Henning RJ: Cocaine: Pathophysiology and clinical toxicology. *Heart Lung* 26(6):466–483, 1997.

Merikle EP: The subjective experience of craving: An exploratory analysis. *Subst Use Misuse* 34(8):1101–1115, 1999.

O'Brien CP: A range of research-based pharmacotherapies for addiction. *Science* 278(5335):66–70, 1997.

PART V

MOOD DISORDERS

15. Depressive Disorders

I **DEPRESSIVE DISORDERS** fall into two major types:

A. Major depression (also known as unipolar depression)
B. Dysthymic disorder

II **MAJOR DEPRESSION**

A. Introduction. Major depression is a serious, relatively common, and sometimes chronic psychiatric disorder. Of patients with severe major depression requiring hospitalization, up to 15% complete suicide. Major depression may also increase the risk of death and disability from medical disorders. Estimates of the **lifetime incidence** of major depression are about **10% in men** and **15% in women.**

B. Clinical manifestations

1. Major depression is a syndrome described by the following criteria, which can be recalled using the memory device of "1,2,3,4,5."

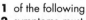

Criteria for major depression (1,2,3,4,5):

1 of the following
2 symptoms must be present for at least **2 weeks:** depressed mood, anhedonia
3 symptoms relating to thought may occur: suicidal ideation, impaired concentration or indecisiveness, guilty preoccupations or feelings of worthlessness
4 physical symptoms: insomnia, decreased energy or fatigue, psychomotor agitation or retardation, weight loss or gain
5 total symptoms must be present

---

2. Major depressive episode refers to a discrete period of symptoms, whereas **depressive disorders** are a diagnostic category. A depressive episode may be part of a major depressive disorder or bipolar disorder (see Chapter 17).

   3. Major depressive episodes may be characterized as having **melancholic, atypical,** or **catatonic features.**

     a. **Melancholic features** are marked by a nearly complete lack of capacity for pleasure, a particular quality to the depressive feelings, early morning awakening, weight loss, psychomotor changes, guilty preoccupations, and depressive feelings that are worse in the morning. **Melancholic depressions tend to be severe, with associated physiologic findings and greater responsiveness to somatic treatments,** and are less likely to be associated with personality disorders. Melancholic features are **more commonly seen in elderly patients.**

     b. **Atypical features** include mood reactivity during the depression, hypersomnia, increased appetite, feelings of "leaden paralysis," and a personality marked by great sensitivity to rejection. This type of depression is more likely to be chronic. **Atypical depressive episodes occur more commonly in younger patients, occur very often in women, and are often associated with personality or anxiety disorders.**

     c. **Catatonic features** indicate characteristic psychomotor disturbances such as mutism, waxy flexibility (catalepsy), stupor, and excessive motor activity.

   4. Psychotic features may occur in the course of severe depressive episodes (see Chapter 9).

   5. Major depressive episodes may also have a seasonal pattern (worse in winter months) or be of postpartum onset.

   6. The average age of onset is 20–40 years of age.

   7. The cultural expression of depression may vary, especially in terms of a tendency to manifest somatic or psychomotor symptoms.

C. Prognosis. If left untreated, depressive episodes may last from 6 months to 2 years. The course of major depressive disorder is variable. Most cases tend to recur; **50%–85% of patients who have one depressive episode will have another.** The pattern of relapse is quite variable. However, the greater the number of prior depressive episodes, the greater the likelihood of subsequent episodes. Five to ten percent of cases may be chronic (lasting more than 2 years). With recurrent depressive episodes, one may or may not have full interepisode recovery.

D. Causes

   1. A deficiency of neurotransmitters, particularly monoamines such as serotonin and norepinephrine, with possible compensatory upregulation of receptors, is thought to underlie symptoms of depression. Antidepressant medications act at this level (see Chapter 16).

   2. Neuroendocrine findings in depressed patients may involve abnormalities in the adrenal gland, thyroid gland, growth hormone, and melatonin system.

   3. Psychological conceptions of depression include aggression turned against the self, learned helplessness, negative cognitive misinterpretations, and overwhelming loss of self-esteem with resultant helplessness.

E. Several **risk factors** for major depression have been established:
  1. A first-degree relative with major depression or with alcohol dependence is a risk factor.
  2. Women are twice as likely to be affected as men.
  3. For women, the 6 months following childbirth is a period of increased risk.
  4. Medical illness and substance abuse may aid in precipitating major depression.
  5. Stressors, particularly losses, may be related to the onset of a major depressive episode, especially earlier in the course of the illness.
  6. Early trauma may play a causative role or affect the expression of depression.

F. **Differential diagnosis**
  1. The differential diagnosis of major depression includes:
    —normal sadness
    —normal bereavement (5% may develop a depressive disorder)
    —adjustment disorders
    —dysthymia (see III)
    —"double depression" (major depression superimposed upon dysthymia)
    —bipolar disorder types I and II (depressive disorders differ from the bipolar disorders in that in depressive disorders there is no history of a manic, mixed manic, or hypomanic episode)
    —schizoaffective disorder, depressed type
    —post-psychotic depression
    —depressive disorder NOS
    —dementia (must be distinguished from "pseudodementia," which refers to the cognitive impairments associated with depression)
    —mood disorder due to a general medical condition (e.g., Parkinson's disease, cerebrovascular accidents, seizure disorders, multiple sclerosis, dementia, head trauma, thyroid disease, adrenal dysfunction, pancreatic carcinoma)
    —substance-induced mood disorder (e.g., as related to illicit drugs, alcohol, or medications including corticosteroids, hormones, antihypertensives, analgesics, central nervous system agents)

HOT ▶ **KEY**

In instances of depression with related alcohol or substance use, the underlying substance use may be an attempt at self-medication of depressive symptoms. Substance use may also cause depressive symptoms. If the latter is true, depressive symptoms will usually remit within 1 month of abstinence.

2. Disorders that coexist with major depression often include:
—substance abuse and dependence
—anxiety disorders including panic disorder (seen in 15%–30% of depressed patients)
—generalized anxiety disorder and obsessive–compulsive disorder
—personality disorders including borderline, obsessive–compulsive, dependent, avoidant, and narcissistic types
—anorexia nervosa and bulimia nervosa

G. Approach to the patient. Patients should be assessed for psychotic symptoms and manic symptoms or a history suggestive of bipolar disorder, as well as for suicidality (see Chapter 7) and potential for aggressive behavior toward others. Remember that the potential for suicide may increase as the patient's energy and motivation are restored with treatment. A full physical examination with relevant laboratory studies should be performed, often including thyroid function tests and a drug screen.

HOT KEY A test of the thyroid-stimulating hormone (TSH) level should **always** be performed on all depressed patients at least once over the course of the illness. This is important because a patient with hypothyroidism may present similarly to one with depression, but the treatment will be different.

H. Treatment

1. Psychotherapy is often used without medication in mild cases of depression or adjunctively with psychopharmacologic treatment in nonresponsive or moderate to severe cases. Psychotherapy may help with symptom relief, coping techniques, addressing associated social or familial difficulties, or resolving underlying unconscious conflicts. Psychotherapy may be particularly indicated if the depressive episode was closely related to a loss or other stressor.

2. Psychoeducation concerning the nature of depression and expectations of treatment can clarify misconceptions, provide hope for the patient, and help enlist the support of the family. For example, a patient for whom an antidepressant has just been prescribed should be educated not to expect optimal antidepressant effects for 4–6 weeks. Without this education, the patient may become discouraged and stop taking the medication prematurely.

3. Antidepressant medication (see Chapter 16).

4. Electroconvulsive therapy (ECT) involves inducing a generalized seizure under anesthesia. It is a safe and effective treatment for depression.

   a. ECT has the advantage of a relatively rapid onset of action. Hence, it should be considered as a first-line treatment for patients with severe psychotic depressions, or potentially dangerous outcomes secondary to severe suicidality or life-threatening catatonia, as well as for patients nonresponsive to medications or who for other reasons require a particularly rapid response.

b. Contraindications to ECT include recent myocardial infarction, some arrhythmias, and intracranial space-occupying lesions.

c. Medical evaluation should include a complete medical history and physical examination with vital signs, complete blood cell (CBC) count, electrolytes, electrocardiogram (EKG), and anesthesia consultation. Antiseizure medications, those that increase seizure threshold, and lithium are typically discontinued or held prior to the treatment.

d. Side effects include postictal confusion and some retrograde and anterograde amnesia. Unilateral rather than bilateral lead placement may limit these side effects but may also limit efficacy.

e. Some patients receive "maintenance ECT" treatments once per month.

5. Light therapy involves daily exposure to a bright, artificial light source. It is sometimes prescribed for depressive disorders with seasonal patterns.

III **DYSTHYMIA** is a chronic low-grade depression. Often, patients do not complain about symptoms unless specifically asked. Dysthymia appears to have a point prevalence of approximately 3%, with women affected two to three times more frequently than men.

A. Clinical manifestations. Dysthymic disorder involves a depressed mood for most days over a 2-year period, never absent for more than 2 months at a stretch, with **two of the six symptoms described below.** The hallmark symptoms of dysthymia are easy to remember using the mnemonic "CHASES" because a good physician always "chases" down the potential diagnosis of dysthymia in a patient who seems sad.

Symptoms of Dysthymia ("CHASES")

Concentration or decision-making ability impaired
Hopeless feelings
Appetite is decreased or increased
Sleep problems—insomnia or hypersomnia
Energy is decreased or fatigue occurs
Self-esteem is decreased

Dysthymia may be seen with atypical features. It tends to present by early adulthood and to follow a chronic course.

B. Risk factors for dysthymia include chronic psychosocial stressors and first-degree relatives with major depression.

C. The **differential diagnosis** of dysthymia is **similar to that of major depressive disorder.** Major depression in partial remission should additionally be considered in the differential diagnosis. Each year, approximately 10% of patients with dysthymia develop major depression, which is called **double depression.** Coexisting disorders may include personality disorders, such as borderline personality disorder, or substance use disorders.

D. Treatment for dysthymia may involve antidepressants or psychotherapy or both (as with major depression).

References

American Psychiatric Association: Practice guidelines for the treatment of patients with major depressive disorder (revision). *Am J Psychiatry* 157(suppl 4):1–45, 2000.

Doris A, Ebmeier K, Shajahan P: Depressive illness. *Lancet* 354(9187):1369–1375, 1999.

16. Antidepressant Medications

I | **INTRODUCTION.** All of the available antidepressants have **equal efficacy.**

A. Response: Two thirds of depressed patients will respond to any given antidepressant, and one third to **placebo.** Patients may respond to placebo because of their hopefulness about the treatment, because of the therapeutic effects of having contact with the treater, or because the natural resolution of symptoms has simply coincided with starting the medication.

B. Choice of medication: Medications should be chosen on the basis of the **features of the depression, side effect profile, history of efficacy** of a particular agent with a particular individual, and **potential drug interactions.**

C. Optimal antidepressant effects may take **4–6 weeks.** Medications should be maintained at least **6–9 months** before tapering is considered unless there is a history of recurrent depressions, in which case **long-term treatment** with antidepressant medication may be indicated.

HOT ▶ **KEY**

All somatic treatments of depression may precipitate mania or hypomania in susceptible individuals.

II | **CLASSES OF ANTIDEPRESSANT MEDICATION**

A. Second-generation antidepressants

1. **Selective serotonin reuptake inhibitors (SSRIs)** have the best-tolerated side effect profile and are relatively safe in overdose. They include **fluoxetine** (Prozac; 20–80 mg/day), **sertraline** (Zoloft; 50–200 mg/day), **paroxetine** (Paxil; 20–60 mg/day), **fluvoxamine** (Luvox; 100–300 mg/day), and **citalopram** (Celexa; 20–40 mg/day). Fluoxetine has the longest half-life (up to 9 days), a relative advantage in patients who may skip doses, but is often activating (i.e., may cause anxiety, agitation, or insomnia). Sertraline is well tolerated by many patients. Paroxetine is the most sedating of this group but has a characteristic withdrawal syndrome of flu-like symptoms when the drug is discontinued. The most common SSRI side effects include gastrointestinal problems (e.g., nausea, vomiting, diarrhea), sexual dysfunction (e.g., de-

creased libido, anorgasmia), weight gain or loss, and sedation or activation.

2. **Bupropion** (Wellbutrin; 300–450 mg/day) is a norepinephrine and dopamine reuptake inhibitor. Bupropion increases the risk of seizure activity, especially when more than 450 mg/day is administered, and may be activating. However, the incidence of sexual side effects may be lower than with other, newer antidepressants.

3. **Venlafaxine** (Effexor; 75–375 mg/day) is a serotonin and norepinephrine reuptake inhibitor (it provides more serotonin blockade at lower doses and more norepinephrine blockade at higher doses). Patients who do not respond adequately to SSRIs may respond to venlafaxine.

4. **Mirtazapine** (Remeron; 15–45 mg/day) is a new antidepressant that enhances both noradrenergic and serotonergic neurotransmission. It may be particularly useful with more severe depression.

5. **Trazodone** (150–500 mg/day) and nefazodone (Serzone; 300–600 mg/day) are related compounds that function as serotonin reuptake inhibitors while also blocking serotonin receptors. Trazodone is a sedating cyclic antidepressant that may induce priapism in men.

B. **Tricyclic antidepressants (TCAs)** block the reuptake of monoamine neurotransmitters. Tricyclic antidepressants include **amitriptyline** (100–300 mg/day), **nortriptyline** (50–200 mg/day), **desipramine** (100–300 mg/day), **clomipramine** (100–250 mg/day), and many others. They are inexpensive and relatively well studied, having been on the market for many years.

1. TCAs may be useful with neuropathic pain.

2. Clomipramine has particular efficacy with obsessive compulsive disorder symptoms.

3. **TCAs have a narrow therapeutic index, and hence blood levels should be followed.** TCAs may have cardiotoxic effects, especially with underlying ventricular arrhythmias, sinus node dysfunction, conduction defects, prolonged QT intervals, or recent myocardial infarction. A baseline electrocardiogram (EKG) should be taken, and consultation with an internist or cardiologist may be indicated if the EKG is abnormal (e.g., conduction delay is present).

4. **TCAs may be associated with weight gain, dry mouth, constipation, blurred vision, and drowsiness.** Because of their anticholinergic activity, caution should be used before prescribing these medications to patients with dementia, narrow-angle glaucoma, or prostate disease. **TCAs may also lead to orthostatic hypotension,** a consideration with elderly patients who may be prone to falling.

HOT ▶ **KEY**   Tricyclic antidepressants can be lethal in overdose.

C. **Monoamine oxidase inhibitors (MAOIs)** block destruction of monoamine neurotransmitters. MAOIs include **isocarboxazid** (10–50 mg/day), **tranylcypromine** (10–40 mg/day), and **phenelzine** (15–90 mg/day). They are a class of antidepressants that have particular efficacy for treatment of **atypical major depression.** As with tricyclics, MAOIs may be associated with weight gain and orthostatic hypotension and, more seriously, **hypertensive crises.** Hence, MAOIs can only be used with patients who can reliably adhere to the **dietary and medication restrictions.** If tyramine-containing foods (e.g., aged cheeses, pickled or smoked meats, yeast, red wine, fava beans) or medications, including sympathomimetics, decongestants, narcotics, and some antihypertensives, are combined with an MAOI, a hypertensive crisis may ensue, leading to sudden severe headache, visual changes, flushing, nausea, and vomiting. **A hypertensive crisis requires emergent medical evaluation and may ultimately be fatal.**

III   **AUGMENTATION STRATEGIES.** Measures to potentiate antidepressant medications include adding **lithium, thyroid hormone** or **stimulants** (e.g., methylphenidate or dextroamphetamine), or mood stabilizers, or **combining antidepressants.** The latter involves close attention to potential toxicities. **The serotonin syndrome is marked by symptoms of tremor, restlessness, myoclonus, hyperthermia, hyperreflexia, hyperpyrexia, hallucinosis, and delirium and may ultimately be fatal.**

HOT ▶ **KEY**   The **serotonin syndrome** may be precipitated by use of two medications with serotonin-enhancing properties (e.g., MAOI with TCA or second-generation antidepressants) or MAOI overdose. A 1–2 week washout period is indicated following TCAs and second-generation antidepressants before starting MAOIs (6 weeks is needed after discontinuing fluoxetine).

References

Nemeroff CB, DeVane CL, Pollack BJ: Newer antidepressants and the cytochrome P450 system. *Am J Psychiatry* 153:311–320, 1996.

Spigset O, Martensson B: Fortnightly review: Drug treatment of depression. *BMJ* 318(7192):1188–1191, 1999.

17. Bipolar Disorders

I INTRODUCTION

A. Bipolar disorders consist of a history of depressive episodes (see Chapter 15) in combination with a history of a manic, mixed manic, or hypomanic episodes (see II).

B. Bipolar disorders include bipolar disorder types I and II, cyclothymia, and bipolar disorder not otherwise specified (NOS).

II MANIC, MIXED MANIC, AND HYPOMANIC EPISODES

A. Criteria for manic episode: elevated, expansive, or irritable mood along with three of the following seven criteria for 1 week or any duration if hospitalization is required (4 weeks if mood is only irritable).

Criteria for manic episode: FLIPPED

Flight of ideas
Less need for sleep
Inflated self-esteem or grandiosity
Pressured speech or more verbally expressive than usual
Psychomotor agitation or increased goal-directed activity
Excessive involvement in pleasurable activities with a high potential for painful consequences (e.g., spending sprees, sexual indiscretion, risky business interactions)
Distractibility

PROFILE

When Mrs. S, who has a longstanding history of bipolar disorder, returned home from an overseas trip, her family noticed that she was sleeping very little and talking with others, including strangers, a great deal. She was animated and silly and making frequent sexual remarks, which was a departure from her usual demeanor. She reported that she "never felt better" and had invested her savings in a new internet business that was going to "make [her] a millionaire." When Mrs. S's family became concerned, because similar symptoms had heralded manic decompensations in the past, she accused them of spying on her and not wanting her to be happy.

B. Criteria for mixed manic episode. In a mixed manic episode, a patient meets criteria for both a manic and a depressive episode simultaneously for 1 week.

C. Hypomanic episodes are similar to manic episodes but may be of shorter duration (at least 4 days). They are not associated with psychosis, or significant impairment, so they rarely require hospitalization.

D. Other characteristics

    1. Rapid cycling refers to at least four mood episodes over a 12-month period. Roughly 10% of patients with bipolar disorder follow this pattern.

    2. As with depressive disorders, bipolar disorders may have catatonic, melancholic, or atypical features; have a postpartum onset; or follow a seasonal pattern (see Chapter 15 II B 3, 4, 5).

III **BIPOLAR DISORDER TYPE I** is a severe and chronic psychiatric illness. The lifetime incidence is 0.5%–1.5% for both men and women. Up to 20% of patients with bipolar I disorder may complete suicide.

A. Clinical manifestations

    1. One or more manic or mixed manic episodes characterize bipolar I disorder. Depressive episodes usually occur as well. Prominent psychotic symptoms are often seen during manic episodes and may be seen during depressive episodes as well.

    2. Untreated, patients may average several episodes per decade with episodes occurring more frequently as the patient's age increases.

    3. For women with bipolar I disorder, the first manifestation of the illness is likely to be a depressive episode, whereas for men it is more likely to be a manic episode.

    4. The onset of the illness typically occurs in late adolescence or early adulthood.

    5. Two thirds of manic episodes immediately precede or follow a depressive episode, often according to a specific pattern for the individual. Cycles tend to occur more quickly as the disorder progresses.

HOT **KEY**
    Up to 30% of patients with bipolar disorder may have functional difficulty between episodes, including mood lability.

B. Causes

    1. Risk factors. Increased rates of bipolar and depressive disorders are seen in first-degree relatives of patients with bipolar disorder. Stressors may be related to the expression of the disorder.

       2. The **kindling theory** proposes that manic episodes kindle further manic episodes. This theory has led to the use of antiseizure medications, such as valproate, carbamazepine, and clonazepam, for bipolar disorder.

       3. Mania may be viewed psychologically as a defensive response to depression.

C. Differential diagnosis and comorbidity

    1. The differential diagnosis for bipolar I disorder includes:

       —substance-induced mood disorder (that which resolves within 1 month of cessation of substance use)

       —mood disorder due to a general medical condition (including thyroid disease, Cushing's disease, cerebral neoplasms)

       —bipolar disorder type II

       —cyclothymic disorder

       —anxiety disorders

       —schizoaffective disorder—bipolar type

       —schizophrenia

       —depressive disorders (especially agitated depressions)

       —attention-deficit hyperactivity disorder (ADHD)

       —borderline personality disorder

       —antisocial personality disorder

       —narcissistic personality disorder

    2. ADHD, substance-related disorders, and anxiety disorders are often comorbid.

D. Approach to the patient. A full psychiatric and medical evaluation should be undertaken at the time of diagnosis and with any change in clinical status. Comorbid or underlying conditions, especially substance use and thyroid disorders, should be treated. The nature of the current episode, including safety and psychotic features, should be assessed, and site of treatment determined. Family history of bipolar disorder suggests that patients with depression are at increased risk for an underlying bipolar disorder.

HOT KEY Denial is a characteristic feature of this disorder. Insight may become more impaired as a patient becomes more manic, and strategies for dealing with this should be developed in advance, ideally through collaboration between the clinician, patient, and family.

E. Treatment

    1. Pharmacological treatment

       a. Mood stabilizers are used to treat manic and depressive episodes and to prevent manic and depressive decompensation, with variable efficacy. Checking for therapeutic levels of a mood stabilizer is often the first step in treating a mood episode. Lithium, valproate, and carbamazepine may be teratogens when used in the first trimester of pregnancy. The **mechanism of action** of lithium seems to be at the level of the second messenger system. Valproate and carbamazepine may act on the gamma-aminobutyric acid (GABA) system.

(1) Lithium (900–2100 mg) may have particular efficacy with classic (euphoric) mania. It may take 2 weeks of administration to reach maximal efficacy during acute mania and 6 weeks during depression. Slow-release forms are available. It is excreted by the kidneys. The half-life is 14–30 hours. Side effects include tremor, sedation, polydipsia and polyuria, gastrointestinal symptoms, cognitive problems, coordination problems, acne, edema, hair loss, weight gain, leukocytosis, cardiac conduction abnormalities, hypothyroidism, and long-term renal effects. Blood urea nitrogen (BUN) and creatinine levels, complete blood cell (CBC) count, thyroid function test (TFT), pregnancy test, and electrocardiogram (EKG) are usually performed at baseline. Lithium levels, electrolytes, and thyroid and renal status should be monitored periodically. Lithium is usually maintained at blood levels of 0.6–0.8 mEq/L for prophylactic use and 0.8–1.2 mEq/L for patients with acute mania.

(2) Valproate (Depakote; 750–3750 mg) may have particular efficacy for patients with mixed manic episodes. It may be administered in loading doses of up to 20 mg/kg. The half-life is 6–16 hours. Side effects include tremor, sedation, gastrointestinal symptoms, hair loss, weight gain, transaminase elevations, leukopenia, and thrombocytopenia. Women begun on valproate before 20 years of age may have significantly increased risk of polycystic ovarian syndrome. Baseline liver function tests (LFTs) and a CBC count should be performed and monitored periodically thereafter. Blood levels are usually maintained at 50–125 mg/L.

(3) Carbamazepine (Tegretol) may have particular efficacy for a patient with rapid cycling. The dosage range begins at 400 mg/day. The side effects of this mood stabilizer may include gastrointestinal symptoms, sedation, dizziness, ataxia, diplopia, hyponatremia, and leukopenia. Baseline laboratory tests include a CBC count with differential and platelets, electrolytes, BUN, creatinine, and LFTs. CBC counts should be followed at regular intervals thereafter. Therapeutic levels of carbamazepine are 8–12 mg/mL.

   (4) Verapamil (320–480 mg). Calcium channel blockers are also used as mood stabilizers. Side effects include hypotension, bradycardia, headache, nausea, and dizziness.

   (5) Lamotrigine (Lamictal; 50–250 mg/day) is a newly marketed anticonvulsant used as a mood stabilizer. Valproate will increase its concentration. Lamotrigine dosage should be increased gradually, and should be stopped if the patient develops a rash.

   (6) Gabapentin (Neurontin) is another newly marketed anticonvulsant used as a mood stabilizer. It is very well tolerated, and it is renally excreted unchanged.

  b. Other medications and combinations. Combinations of mood stabilizers, or mood stabilizers with benzodiazepines or antipsychotic agents, are used to control acute manic symptoms because mood stabilizers may take 2–3 weeks to reach maximal efficacy. When combinations of mood stabilizers are used, particular attention must be paid to interactions. Antidepressants may be combined with antipsychotics or mood stabilizers.

HOT

 All antidepressants may "flip" a bipolar depressed patient into mania and so should be used with great caution.

KEY

---

 2. Electroconvulsive therapy (ECT) may be used to treat both the depressive and manic phases of bipolar disorder.

 3. Psychotherapeutic treatment

  a. Between acute episodes, patients and families should be educated about the nature of bipolar illness and the patient should be helped to understand his or her own characteristic signs of decompensation. The importance of regular sleep patterns and maintenance medications should be addressed.

  b. Psychotherapeutic goals should be gauged to individual circumstances but may involve learning to limit or manage stressors.

 BIPOLAR DISORDER TYPE II is marked by at least one depressive and one hypomanic episode. Usually, the mood is elevated and the patient may be more social or productive. The differential diagnosis and comorbid conditions are similar to those of bipolar I disorder. Bipolar II disorder occurs more frequently in women than men. Its lifetime incidence is 0.5%.

It may also present in a rapid-cycling form. Episodes occur less frequently as the patient's age increases. Patients seem to be at increased risk if there is a first-degree relative with bipolar or major depressive disorder. Treatment may involve use of mood stabilizers and antidepressants.

 CYCLOTHYMIC DISORDER is marked by multiple episodes of hypomanic and depressive symptoms; however, the symptoms are not at the level of a major depression or full manic episode. Treatment may involve use of mood stabilizers and antidepressants.

References

Akiskal HS, Pinto O: The evolving bipolar spectrum: Prototype I, II, III, and IV. *Psychiatr Clin North Am* 22(3):517, 1999.

The Expert Consensus Guideline Series: Treatment of bipolar disorder. *J Clin Psychiatry* 57(suppl 12A), 1996.

Hilty DM, Brady KT, Hales RE: A review of bipolar disorder among adults. *Psychiatr Serv* 50(2):201–213, 1999.

Kilzieh N, Akiskal HS: Rapid-cycling bipolar disorder: An overview of research and clinical experience. *Psychiatr Clin North Am* 22(3):585, 1999.

PART VI

ANXIETY DISORDERS

18. Panic and Generalized Anxiety Disorders

I **INTRODUCTION.** Anxiety is a normal response to a stressful situation and may be caused by many different factors. Everyone feels anxious sometimes. However, some people feel anxious all the time.

A. Anxiety is considered **pathological** when the symptoms are so overwhelming that they **clearly impair a person's ability to work, socialize,** or **enjoy life.**

B. Anxiety may arise **spontaneously,** as a primary anxiety disorder, or it may be triggered by **another psychiatric disorder or an underlying medical condition.**

HOT KEY Primary anxiety disorders are very common, affecting approximately 10%–15% of the population at some point in their lifetime.

II **CLINICAL MANIFESTATIONS.** Anxiety presents in many forms clinically, and some anxiety disorders have symptoms in common. Anxiety may be **constant and generalized** or may cause very **discrete episodes of panic,** among other presentations. Some people have both types. **Unexpected episodes** of anxiety are the norm, although **specific events or objects** may trigger bouts of intense discomfort.

A. Generalized anxiety disorder (GAD)

1. GAD causes overwhelming worry, fear, or apprehension. Patients may feel anxious and may even state what they think is the cause (e.g., they can't seem to get their minds off real-life worries). They may also complain of difficulty concentrating or of their minds going "blank."

2. These patients have persistent feelings of being "keyed up." They may feel tense and restless, and signs of autonomic arousal (e.g., rapid heartbeat, sweating) may be evident.

   3. The patient may be hypervigilant (i.e., constantly "scanning" their surroundings for the "cause" of their anxious feelings).
   4. A diagnosis of GAD is made when these symptoms occur more days than not for at least 6 months and when the anxiety is not specific to any one event or situation. Often, related symptoms (e.g., problems with sleep, loss of appetite) are also present.
B. Panic attacks
   1. Definition. A **panic attack** is a **sudden, unexpected episode of intense fear** that is accompanied by at least four of the following symptoms:
      a. Palpitations
      b. Sweating
      c. Trembling or shaking
      d. Shortness of breath
      e. Chest pain or discomfort
      f. Choking
      g. Numbness or tingling
      h. Chills or hot flashes
      i. Nausea or abdominal distress
      j. Dizziness or light-headedness
      k. Derealization (feelings of unreality) or depersonalization (feeling detached from oneself)
      l. Fear of losing control or of "going crazy"
      m. Fear of dying
   2. Duration. Panic attacks usually last 5–30 minutes. The symptoms peak in the first 10 minutes. These episodes can be triggered by specific situations, but they usually occur with no warning. This tendency makes them even more frightening. They may occur at any time and may even awaken people from sleep.
   3. Risk of misdiagnosis. Some people mistake the physical manifestations of anxiety for a medical problem, especially if the symptoms take the form of a panic attack. **An isolated panic attack does not constitute an anxiety disorder,** but a number of anxiety disorders have panic attacks as part of the syndrome.
C. Panic disorder. When a person has repeated panic episodes for at least 1 month and begins to fearfully anticipate having another attack, the anxiety has become panic disorder.

HOT KEY Uncontrolled panic disorder is very disabling: 70% of people with this disorder lose or quit their jobs, and 50% will not drive farther than a few miles from home.

D. Agoraphobia. A person who has panic symptoms often attempts to flee the situation and to avoid similar situations. Agoraphobia is an **intense fear of being in situations where escape might be difficult.** The pattern of avoidance may generalize to such an extent that the patient is afraid to venture out of the house. People who have agoraphobia may venture out of their homes only with companions, or they may avoid situations and places that limit their ability to escape (e.g., highways) or places where crowds and lines are expected (e.g., public transportation, busy stores).

III **CAUSES.** Several mechanisms in the brain contribute to the symptoms of apprehension, worry, and fear. Some or all of these brain mechanisms may be overactive in patients with GAD and panic disorders.

A. Norepinephrine neurons that project from the locus ceruleus become hypersensitive and cause cortical activation as well as peripheral autonomic effects (e.g., tremor, sweating, tachycardia, dilated pupils).
B. When activated by benzodiazepines, gamma-aminobutyric acid (GABA) receptors in the cortex decrease apprehension. Some people may be particularly susceptible to anxiety because they lack a putative endogenous benzodiazepine-like substance.
C. Excess release of **serotonin** in the frontal and limbic regions promotes anxious feelings.

IV **APPROACH TO THE PATIENT.** Panic attacks are a frequent cause of visits to the emergency department. Anxiety is never comfortable, so it is important to **be calm and empathetic** with the patient. To help clarify the type of anxiety disorder the patient has, the clinician should try to find out:

A. What, if anything, provokes anxiety
B. How intense the anxiety is and how quickly it develops
C. What physical symptoms accompany the anxiety
D. What, if anything, makes the anxiety better (e.g., social isolation vs. companionship)
E. How long the symptoms have been present and the nature of their progression
F. What situations the patient avoids to minimize the symptoms
G. How much the patient's life is impaired by the avoidance and the anxiety symptoms
H. What medications and medical or other psychiatric illnesses are present

V **DIFFERENTIAL DIAGNOSIS.** Many psychiatric disorders have panic attacks associated with them. The key distinguishing feature of panic disorder is **unexpected panic attacks.**

A. **Panic disorder** usually causes multiple unexpected panic attacks.

B. **Posttraumatic stress disorder, social phobia,** and **specific phobia** are associated with panic episodes on exposure to a feared stimulus or situation.

C. **GAD** is characterized by nearly constant high levels of anxiety rather than by discrete episodes of panic. Patients with GAD may also have superimposed panic attacks. In addition, many people who have GAD have comorbid major depression. The rate of suicide is dramatically increased in these patients.

D. **Underlying medical problems** also may cause symptoms of autonomic arousal (e.g., palpitations, flushing) and must be distinguished from anxiety. These conditions include:
   1. Hypoglycemia (and insulinoma)
   2. Hyperthyroidism
   3. Hypoxemia due to any cause (e.g., chronic obstructive pulmonary disease, congestive heart failure)
   4. Pheochromocytoma (because of catecholamine secretion)
   5. Acute intermittent porphyria
   6. Myocardial ischemia or infarction

E. **Many medications and drugs** also cause anxiety, including:
   1. Caffeine
   2. Nicotine
   3. Stimulants, including cocaine
   4. Theophylline and β-agonists

F. **Withdrawal from alcohol or sedatives** (especially short-acting hypnotic agents) can also cause anxiety.

VI **TREATMENT.** Fortunately, there are many effective treatments for anxiety disorders. Usually, a **combination of medication and therapy** is helpful.

A. **Reassurance.** It is very important to start the treatment with an explanation of the nature of anxiety (i.e., the patient's brain is making them feel as though they are in danger when, in reality, they are not). Even if a thorough evaluation finds no medical cause for the symptoms, the patient may still feel worried that something was missed. In this case, it is important to reassure the patient that the symptoms are real and are generated by an imbalance of brain chemicals.

B. **Substance abuse.** It is important to ask about abuse of alcohol, marijuana, or other substances that the patient may use to temporarily alleviate anxiety. Long-term abuse of alcohol or marijuana invariably worsens the symptoms of anxiety and can also cause mood and sleep disturbances.

HOT KEY Don't make the mistake of telling the patient "it's all in your head"—even if the patient says this. There are better ways to explain what is happening clinically.

C. Therapy

1. **Cognitive-behavioral therapy** is very effective for treating both GAD and panic disorder. This therapy teaches the patients to focus on thoughts and behaviors that they have in anticipation of anxiety or panic episodes so that they can learn alternate, more helpful thought and behavior patterns.
2. **Relaxation training** is helpful to teach the patient how to achieve control of the physiologic arousal that accompanies anxiety. Progressive relaxation and abdominal breathing techniques are often used, sometimes in combination with biofeedback.

D. Medications

1. **Anxiolytics**
   a. **Highly potent benzodiazepines** are most effective for panic disorder (e.g., alprazolam 0.25–0.50 mg orally 3 times daily, increased by 0.25–0.50 every 2–3 days to a final dose of 2–6 mg/day in divided doses; or clonazepam 0.25–0.50 orally twice daily, increased by 0.25–0.50 every 3–5 days until the patient is maintained on 1–3 mg/day).
   b. **All benzodiazepines** are effective for GAD (e.g., diazepam 5–10 mg orally 3–4 times daily). Tolerance develops to the side effects within a few weeks, but tolerance rarely develops to the antianxiety effects.
   c. **β-Blockers** are useful for decreasing the autonomic effects of anxiety, but they do not relieve the anticipatory anxiety. For performance anxiety, the patient should be given propranolol 10–40 mg orally a half hour before the event. Make sure to try a test dose before the important event. These drugs are contraindicated in patients who have heart block, bradycardia, asthma, or diabetes.

2. **Antidepressants**
   a. **Selective serotonin reuptake inhibitors (SSRIs)** are very effective in the treatment of panic disorder and other anxiety disorders. To avoid initially exacerbating the anxious feelings, it is important to start with very low doses and titrate up slowly [e.g., 5 mg paroxetine (Paxil) or fluoxetine (Prozac) orally every day: increase by 5 mg every 5–7 days to 20 mg, and then increase 10–20 mg every 4 weeks

until symptoms remit; 25 mg sertraline (Zoloft) or fluvox-amine (Luvox): increase 25 mg every 5–7 days to 100 mg, and increase 50 mg if no improvement is seen after 4 weeks, to a maximum dose of 200 mg].

b. Tricyclic antidepressants (TCAs) such as imipramine or amitriptyline are effective for panic disorder and sometimes also for GAD (e.g., start with 50 mg imipramine or 25 mg amitriptyline at bedtime, and titrate up 50 or 25 mg, respectively, every week, to 150–200 mg at bedtime or until symptoms remit).

c. Venlafaxine is very effective for GAD. Start with 37.5 mg orally twice daily (or 75 mg of the extended-release form) and increase by 75 mg/day every 2–4 weeks. It is important to monitor blood pressure during treatment because sustained hypertension occasionally results.

VII FOLLOW-UP AND REFERRAL

A. GAD is often chronic and requires long-term treatment. However, many people feel anxiety-free with medications and effective therapy.

B. Panic disorder is likely to remit with proper treatment.

C. Referral for substance abuse treatment is necessary for patients who rely on alcohol, marijuana, or other drugs.

References

Leaman TL: Anxiety disorders. *Prim Care* 26(2):197–210, 1999.

Sheehan DV: Current concepts in the treatment of panic disorder. *J Clin Psychiatry* 60(suppl 18):16–21, 1999.

Sullivan GM, Coplan JD, Kent JM, et al: The noradrenergic system in pathological anxiety: A focus on panic with relevance to generalized anxiety and phobias. *Biol Psychiatry* 46(9):1205–1218, 1999.

19. Phobias

I **INTRODUCTION.** Sometimes **anxiety** is triggered by **specific situations, events, or objects.** Patients with phobias may experience **discrete episodes of panic** or may have a **more generalized feeling of anxiety.** The keys to these disorders are what stimulus provokes the anxiety and how the patient's life is affected by trying to avoid the stimulus.

II **CLINICAL MANIFESTATIONS**

A. **Social phobia,** or **social anxiety disorder,** is an intense fear of social situations because of the potential for **embarrassment** or **perceived scrutiny by others.** Patients with social phobia may even fear casual conversations with a friend.

B. **Specific phobia** is an irrational fear of a **specific situation, activity, or object.** The focus of the phobia may evoke either generalized or panic forms of anxiety. The fear may become so intense that efforts to avoid the feared object or event cause significant disruption in the person's life. The most common phobias are of **animals, blood** or **needles, heights** (acrophobia), and **small or crowded spaces** (claustrophobia). Unlike most other anxiety disorders, specific phobias usually develop during the preadolescent years.

III **CAUSES.** Phobias often develop as a result of an **initially intense anxious feeling in association with a specific stimulus** (i.e., a form of classical conditioning). For instance, a person who has an especially strong vasovagal response may have a phobia of needles or blood after being frightened by nearly passing out during a blood test. In susceptible individuals, the initially frightening experience is amplified to the point of panic or near-panic when a similar experience occurs. Some people may be especially susceptible to these types of responses because their **brain mechanisms for handling anxiety are especially sensitive** (see Chapter 18 III).

IV **APPROACH TO THE PATIENT.** Obtaining a history that identifies the focus of a phobia is usually straightforward, unless the patient is especially embarrassed by the symptoms. People who have social phobia may even avoid treatment settings because they have a fear of interacting with people. In taking a history, it is important to focus on:

A. What, if anything, provokes the anxiety
B. How intense the anxiety is and how quickly it develops
C. What physical symptoms accompany the anxiety
D. What, if anything, makes the anxiety better (e.g., social isolation vs. companionship)
E. How long the symptoms have been present and their progression
F. What situations the patient avoids to minimize the symptoms (e.g., elevators, travel)
G. How much the patient's life is impaired by avoiding certain places or situations as well as by the anxiety symptoms
H. What medications and medical or other psychiatric illnesses are present

V DIFFERENTIAL DIAGNOSIS

A. Social phobia must be distinguished from agoraphobia. People with **agoraphobia** are afraid to venture out alone. They are re-assured by having people around to turn to in case of panic symptoms. People with **social phobia** will venture out alone without anxiety as long as they are reasonably certain that they will not encounter a social situation.
B. The tendency of people with social phobia to isolate may also make them appear to have a **depressive disorder.** It is important to perform a thorough evaluation to assess this possibility.
C. People with **schizotypal personality disorder** may have exces-sive anxiety about social encounters, but they also are usually excessively paranoid or bizarre.

VI TREATMENT

A. Therapy
  1. **"Graded exposure"** to the feared stimulus is a behavioral therapy that uses increasing exposure to objects or events, leading up to the most feared. For instance, first talking about a feared situation (e.g., heights), then visualizing it or looking at pictures of it, then finally encountering the situa-tion. Relaxation techniques are incorporated at each step to counter the anxiety symptoms.
  2. **Eye movement desensitization and reprocessing (EMDR)** uses guided eye movements during imagined exposure to feared stimuli to reduce the fearfulness.
  3. **Group therapy** is a form of graded exposure for social pho-bia. Severely anxious patients may require individual treat-ment first.
B. Medications
  1. No medications are known to be effective for treating spe-cific phobias. In contrast, there are some very effective med-

ications for social phobia. For panic and general feelings of anxiety that accompany phobic disorders, use medications as described in Chapter 18.

2. For acutely anxious patients, **high-potency benzodiazepines** are the treatment of choice (e.g., lorazepam 0.5–1.0 mg orally every 4 hours; alprazolam 0.25–0.50 mg orally every 6 hours; or clonazepam 0.25–0.50 orally twice daily) until the anxiety is under control. It is best to use the lowest dose that provides adequate relief of symptoms.

3. Several **antidepressants** are effective in treating the symptoms of social phobia:

   a. **Selective serotonin reuptake inhibitors (SSRIs)** [i.e., paroxetine, fluoxetine, sertraline, or fluvoxamine] are administered at the same doses as in GAD and panic disorder (see Chapter 18 VI D 2 a).

   b. **Monoamine oxidase inhibitors (MAOIs)** [e.g., phenelzine: start with 30 mg orally every day, and increase by 15 mg every 4 weeks until symptoms remit (maximum dose 90 mg)]. Remember to advise the patient to strictly avoid tyramine-rich foods.

   c. **Tricyclic antidepressants (TCAs)** (e.g., imipramine or amitriptyline) are administered at the same doses as in GAD and panic disorder (see Chapter 18 VI D 2 b).

VII **FOLLOW-UP AND REFERRAL.** Phobic disorders can be greatly debilitating. Proper follow-up treatment is needed because these disorders are usually chronic. After the symptoms are controlled, periodic reassessment and treatment may be needed to sustain remission.

References

Beidel DC: Social anxiety disorder: Etiology and early clinical presentation. *J Clin Psychiatry* (suppl 17):27–32, 1998.

Davidson JR: Pharmacotherapy of social anxiety disorder. *J Clin Psychiatry* (suppl 17):47–53, 1998.

De Jongh A, Ten Broeke E, Renssen MR: Treatment of specific phobias with eye movement desensitization and reprocessing (EMDR): Protocol, empirical status, and conceptual issues. *J Anxiety Disord* 13(1–2):69–85, 1999.

Fyer AJ: Current approaches to etiology and pathophysiology of specific phobia. *Biol Psychiatry* 44(12):1295–1304, 1998.

Otto MW: Cognitive-behavioral therapy for social anxiety disorder: Model, methods, outcome. *J Clin Psychiatry* (suppl 9):14–19, 1999.

20. Acute and Posttraumatic Stress Disorder

I **INTRODUCTION.** In the face of an **overwhelmingly stressful event,** people can experience severe anxiety symptoms. If these anxiety symptoms are not treated rapidly, persistent debilitating anxiety symptoms may occur in the form of **posttraumatic stress disorder (PTSD).**

II **CLINICAL MANIFESTATIONS**

A. **Acute stress disorder** involves a mixture of anxiety symptoms that develop in a person who has experienced or witnessed a severe trauma (e.g., car accident, assault, hurricane). Intense fear, horror, or helplessness follows the person's traumatic experience. Within hours to days of the event, the following symptoms occur and last up to a month:
   1. **Dissociative symptoms** (at least three of these occur):
      a. A sense of numbing or detachment
      b. Being dazed or unaware of surroundings
      c. Feelings of derealization
      d. Feelings of depersonalization
      e. Dissociative amnesia—an inability to recall an important aspect of the trauma
   2. **Recurrent images, thoughts, dreams, or illusions** of reliving the experience
   3. **Avoidance of stimuli** that may arouse memories of the event
   4. **Marked symptoms of anxiety or increased arousal** (e.g., exaggerated startle response, restlessness, difficulty sleeping)
B. When these symptoms last longer than a month, the diagnosis is **PTSD.** The characteristics of PTSD can be easily remembered using the mnemonic "VIETNAM" (because, unfortunately, many Vietnam veterans have PTSD)

III **CAUSES.** These disorders are precipitated by the **traumatic event** itself. One theory about acute stress disorder is that the traumatic event "overloads" the person's normal pathways for handling anxiety. Later, when the person remembers the event or experiences a similar situation, the overstimulated circuits are reactivated, and the symptoms of PTSD (e.g., flashbacks, numbing, panic) occur. For example, a soldier may have horrific

Common characteristics of PTSD ("VIETNAM")

Vigilance increased, along with other generalized or panic-like anxiety symptoms
Intrusive thoughts or images of the event
Experiencing the event in recurring flashbacks
Trauma-related stimuli are avoided
Numbing or emotional detachment
Amnesia for important parts of the traumatic event
Month or more of the above symptoms

memories of being trapped in the trenches with a buddy who got blown up beside him. Later on, any crowded space or sudden, loud noise may evoke a flashback of this powerful and devastating experience. Some patients may have hypersensitivity of the underlying brain mechanisms that create the experience of panic, apprehension, and motor tension (see Chapter 18 III).

IV APPROACH TO THE PATIENT

A. Acute stress disorders may present in the midst of **crisis from the precipitating event.** It is important to be **calm and empathetic** with the patient. Try to obtain as much information from the patient as possible. You may also need to rely on **family members or others involved in the trauma.** Information obtained from others will help to clarify what the patient has experienced and can guide some aspects of treatment.

B. Even though the traumatic event may have occurred some time (even many years) ago, patients with PTSD may **feel as though the traumatic event just happened** because their brain keeps making them relive it, especially if a **more current stressor** has reactivated old symptoms.

C. Both acute stress disorder and PTSD require a careful patient assessment to obtain the whole story. It is important to focus on:
1. What the patient recalls of the incident
2. What anxiety symptoms have developed
3. What physical symptoms accompany the anxiety
4. What, if anything, makes the anxiety better
5. What situations the patient avoids to minimize the symptoms
6. How much the patient's life is impaired by the avoidance and the anxiety symptoms (e.g., diminished interest in activities, feeling detached from people)
7. What sleep problems are present (e.g., sleeplessness, panic, nightmares)

V **DIFFERENTIAL DIAGNOSIS.** Usually, there is no mistaking the source of anxiety in people who have experienced trauma. What can be confusing is the number of different symptoms present, from emotional numbing and social withdrawal to clear-cut panic episodes. It may also be difficult to relate current symptoms to a traumatic event that took place years ago. Intrusive recollection of a traumatic experience may be confused with psychotic hallucinations or delusions.

HOT

KEY

Be sure to evaluate patients for comorbid depressive disorders, especially if suicidal ideation or hopelessness is evident. It is also important to screen these patients carefully for underlying substance abuse, which can precipitate or aggravate mood and anxiety symptoms.

VI **TREATMENT**

A. Therapy for acute stress disorder. An acute reaction to stress warrants **immediate clinical attention** to help the patient process the event emotionally. Otherwise, severe, chronic symptoms of PTSD may develop. The clinician should:

1. Allow the patient to **tell the story.**
2. Provide **emotional support** and encourage the patient to **accept what has happened.**
3. **Provide reality testing** and discuss the nature of the accident, how the situation was handled, and the time frame. From collateral sources (e.g., emergency medical services crew, family members), you may be able to help the patient understand the "bigger picture" of the trauma. For instance, knowing that there was no way of preventing the collision because of the road condition, other driver, or faulty brakes, the patient may assume less guilt about the outcome of a car accident.

B. Agitated or sleepless patients may benefit from the use of a **sedative-hypnotic** (see VI D). The patient should be educated about avoiding use of alcohol or other substances.

C. Therapy for PTSD

1. **Eye movement desensitization and reprocessing (EMDR)** is an effective technique for treating PTSD. The therapist elicits a series of specific eye movements while guiding the patient through emotionally charged memories. The process appears to take the "charge" out of memories, thereby reducing flashbacks and anxiety levels.

2. **Relaxation training** can help the patient to control the physiologic arousal that accompanies anxiety.

3. **Group therapy** is useful for patients who have experienced trauma (e.g., war, rape). These patients obtain support from people with similar experiences.

D. Medications

1. For acutely anxious patients, **high-potency benzodiazepines** are the treatment of choice (e.g., lorazepam 0.5–2.0 mg orally every 4 hours; alprazolam 0.25–1.0 mg orally every 6 hours; or clonazepam 0.25–1.0 orally twice daily) until anxiety is under control. It is best to use the lowest dose that provides adequate relief of symptoms.

2. **Selective serotonin reuptake inhibitors (SSRIs)** are used to treat panic or generalized anxiety symptoms that accompany PTSD. To avoid initially exacerbating the anxious feelings, start with very low doses and titrate up slowly [e.g., 5 mg paroxetine (Paxil) or fluoxetine (Prozac) orally every day: increase by 5 mg every 5–7 days to 20 mg, and then increase 10–20 mg every 4 weeks until symptoms remit; 25 mg sertraline (Zoloft) or fluvoxamine (Luvox) daily by mouth: increase by 25 mg every 5–7 days to 100 mg, and increase 50 mg if no improvement is seen after 4 weeks, to a maximum dose of 200 mg].

3. **Tricyclic antidepressants (TCAs)** are also effective in treating PTSD (see Chapter 18 VI D 2 b for dosages).

4. **Monoamine oxidase inhibitors** are also useful for PTSD [e.g., phenelzine: start with 30 mg orally every day and increase by 15 mg every 4 weeks until symptoms remit (maximum dose 90 mg)]. Remember to advise the patient to strictly avoid tyramine-rich foods.

VII FOLLOW-UP AND REFERRAL

A. Patients who have **acute stress disorder** need a clear follow-up plan.

1. Make sure that **appropriate medications** are dispensed to help the patient manage overwhelming anxiety or sleeplessness.

2. Refer the patient to a clinician who is skilled in **crisis counseling.**

3. If appropriate, refer the patient to a group for **further supportive treatment.**

B. PTSD usually requires **long-term treatment.** These patients may require a number of clinical modalities, such as individual behavioral treatment, group therapy, and substance abuse treatment.

References

Breslau N, Peterson EL, Kessler RC, et al: Short screening scale for DSM-IV post-traumatic stress disorder. *Am J Psychiatry* 156(6):908–911, 1999.

Vaughan K, Armstrong MS, Gold R, et al: A trial of eye movement desensitization compared to image habituation training and applied muscle relaxation in post-traumatic stress disorder. *J Behav Ther Exp Psychiatry* 25:283–291, 1994.

21. Obsessive–Compulsive Disorder

I **INTRODUCTION.** One of the most striking forms of anxiety is the constellation of symptoms known as **obsessive–compulsive disorder (OCD).** Until recently, OCD was considered a rare disorder, but it is now clear that OCD is a **common illness,** with a lifetime prevalence of 2%–3%.

HOT KEY OCD is considered an anxiety disorder because the symptoms (i.e., obsessions and compulsions) are largely driven by internal, overwhelming anxiety.

II **CLINICAL MANIFESTATIONS**

A. According to DSM-IV, the diagnosis of OCD requires that a person have either **obsessions or compulsions** that the patient recognizes as **unreasonable or excessive** and that cause **significant distress** or **impair the patient's life** in some fundamental way.

B. Obsessions

1. Obsessions are **recurrent thoughts, images, or impulses** that are **intrusive and unwanted.** These obsessions cause patients with OCD significant distress, even though these patients clearly recognize that the obsessions are coming from their own mind.

2. These thoughts or impulses are not simply overwhelming real-life worries.

3. **Attempts to ignore these thoughts** or images do not work. Instead, compulsions, which are attempts to suppress the intrusive thought or impulse with another thought or action, develop.

4. The **most common obsessions** are repetitive thoughts of **violence** (e.g., killing one's child), **doubt** (e.g., worrying that the stove was left on), or **contamination** (e.g., worrying that touching someone will result in a terrible disease).

C. Compulsions

1. Compulsions are behaviors that the person feels **driven to perform (usually repeatedly),** in a specific, rigid way in response to an obsession.

   2. Although the person with OCD understands that the compulsion cannot realistically change events, the compulsive behavior is believed to prevent a dreaded event. Therefore, the compulsive behavior relieves the anxiety symptoms, at least temporarily.
   3. The **most common compulsions** are **checking, counting, washing hands,** and **placing items in order.** Compulsions are also called **rituals** because they are repeated so often in exactly the same way (e.g., lock and unlock the door five times, step outside, and repeat).

III **CAUSES.** Rarely, OCD occurs after a traumatic injury to the brain. It usually arises spontaneously in children or young adults (most patients are symptomatic by 25 years of age). Several factors may contribute to the development of OCD.

A. Genetic factors. Patients with OCD are at increased risk for motor tics and Tourette's disorder. All of these disorders run in families.
B. Neurotransmitter activity. The balance of activity in the serotonin system and perhaps the adrenergic system appears to be fundamental to this disorder.
C. Psychodynamic theories. Some people find their normal aggressive impulses unacceptable. In these people, the healthy defense mechanisms may have gone awry. These patients experience so much anxiety that the pathological coping mechanisms of obsessions or compulsions result.

IV **APPROACH TO THE PATIENT**

A. The symptoms of OCD are sometimes dramatic (e.g., patient cannot leave the rest room for 2 hours because of excessive hand washing). More often, however, patients hide their symptoms because they recognize their behavior as excessive and are embarrassed by it. The following checklist is a "review of systems" for OCD symptoms:
   1. How many times do you check things before you leave the house?
   2. Are you ever late because it took you so long to check things?
   3. How often do you find yourself repeating your actions?
   4. Do you tend to count things?
   5. Do you feel concerned about germs and disease?
   6. How long do you spend washing (e.g., hands, feet, household objects)?
   7. Are you ever bothered by unpleasant thoughts that keep returning?

  8. Do you feel compelled to organize, sort, or arrange things?
  9. Do you have trouble completing tasks because you devote so much time to details?
  10. How often do you feel that something you've done carefully is not quite right?

B. If the patient's response to any of these questions is affirmative or seems to identify excessive activity in one area, make sure to explore the topic further. Ask the patient to describe her thoughts and feelings about the compulsive behavior. How distressing are they? Ask how long the rituals took in the past, and how long they take now. In what ways do the obsessions or compulsions interfere with the patient's life? Does the patient feel that he has any control over the rituals, and if so, how?

HOT KEY Be sure to ask the patient about mood and anxiety symptoms. Patients with OCD often have depressive disorders, panic, or generalized anxiety symptoms, which often complicates treatment.

V DIFFERENTIAL DIAGNOSIS

A. Obsessive–compulsive personality disorder may be confused with OCD. Occasionally, the two disorders overlap, although people with OCD usually do not have the all-encompassing character traits that define the personality disorder. The obsessions and compulsions that occur with OCD arise independent of the patient's baseline personality structure (see Chapter 23 II D 3 a).

B. Phobic disorders must be distinguished from OCD, especially phobias about blood, dirt, or contamination. Both patients with phobias and those with OCD avoid the feared object or situation. However, only patients with OCD experience obsessions or engage in ritualistic compulsive behavior.

C. Patients with **schizophrenia** sometimes exhibit behavior that is compulsive, but usually only in response to a **delusion.** Patients with OCD may have an obsession that is so overvalued that it seems almost delusional. However, with further exploration, the patient with OCD can usually acknowledge that these fears are unrealistic. Patients who have schizophrenia often have other psychotic symptoms that clarify the diagnosis.

D. Tourette's disorder is a syndrome of **chronic, multiple motor and vocal tics** (e.g., shouting obscenities). The patient experiences these tics as unavoidable. These patients can suppress the tics for a time, but the movements and vocalizations eventually occur. The absence of obsessive thoughts helps to distinguish Tourette's disorder from OCD. However, many patients with

Tourette's disorder have OCD, and approximately 20% of patients with OCD exhibit motor tics.

E. Body dysmorphic disorder is a somatoform disorder characterized by preoccupation with an **imagined defect in physical appearance.** The imagined defect is clearly out of proportion to the real anomaly. People with this disorder often make repeated attempts to correct or conceal the defect (e.g., cosmetic surgery), but the attempt rarely improves the patient's feelings of disfigurement. The persistence of intrusive thoughts about the defect may dominate the clinical presentation. However, unlike OCD, in which the patient understands that his or her concerns are unrealistic, people with body dysmorphic disorder insist that their worries are justified.

HOT

KEY

Body dysmorphic disorder is common among patients with OCD.

VI **TREATMENT.** Medication in combination with behavior therapy is the treatment of choice. Some patients respond well to medication or behavior therapy alone, but others do not respond at all.

A. Behavior therapy. The patient is subjected to real or imagined exposure to feared stimuli but prevented from performing ritual behaviors. This therapy usually produces **a change in the rituals but not the obsessions.**

B. Medications

1. **Selective serotonin reuptake inhibitors (SSRIs)** are often required at high doses to evoke a response (e.g., fluvoxamine: titrate up to 300 mg/day; paroxetine: up to 60 mg/day; or fluoxetine: up to 80 mg/day).

2. **Tricyclic antidepressants (TCAs).** Clomipramine (titrate up to 250 mg/day) is particularly efficacious, but most of the other TCAs are also effective.

3. **Monoamine oxidase inhibitors (MAOIs)** are especially helpful for patients who have comorbid panic or severe anxiety (e.g., phenelzine 30–90 mg/day).

4. **Antipsychotics.** The atypical antipsychotic risperidone (e.g., 0.5–3 mg at bedtime) may augment the effect of antidepressants that are used to treat OCD but evoke only a partial response.

C. Psychosurgery. A surgical procedure to cut fibers in the cingulate gyrus (cingulotomy) may be effective for severe OCD that is resistant to other forms of treatment. Recent developments allow this procedure to be performed selectively with few complications. However, patients often reexperience symptoms a few weeks or months after the operation.

 FOLLOW-UP AND REFERRAL. OCD is usually a **chronic illness** that requires **long-term treatment.** Patients with OCD may need to be referred to a clinician who is experienced in all modes of standard treatment, including behavior therapy. Psychodynamic psychotherapy alone is not an appropriate follow-up treatment.

References

Goodman WK: Obsessive–compulsive disorder: Diagnosis and treatment. *J Clin Psychiatry* 60(18):27–32, 1999.

Khouzam HR: Obsessive–compulsive disorder. What to do if you recognize baffling behavior. *Postgrad Med* 106(7):133–141, 1999.

Phillips KA, Gunderson CG, Mallya G, et al: A comparison study of body dysmorphic disorder and obsessive-compulsive disorder. *J Clin Psychiatry* 59(11):568–575, 1998.

PART VII

DISSOCIATIVE DISORDERS

22. Dissociative Disorders

I **INTRODUCTION.** Dissociation is a **split between conscious awareness and disturbing memories or feelings.** This splitting process can affect memory and behavior and therefore can present clinically in a number of ways. Dissociative processes usually begin as an **extreme form of psychological defense** against unbearable feelings or memories. Dissociative disorders may evolve when patients continue to use these defenses, even when they are no longer needed.

II **CLINICAL MANIFESTATIONS.** The process of dissociation is similar to hypnosis: For some period of time, **conscious awareness of the self is altered** in a way that causes amnesia or affects personal identity. Three important clinical syndromes may result: dissociative amnesia, dissociative fugue, and dissociative identity disorder.

A. **Dissociative amnesia**
   1. Dissociative amnesia is an **abrupt loss of memory of one or more personal experiences.** These experiences are often **physically or emotionally traumatic events.**
   2. The patient **cannot recall** any events that occurred during a specific period of time, usually before, during, and after a traumatic event.
   3. The amnestic period may be hours, days, or rarely, the patient's entire life.
   4. The memory loss affects only **explicit memory of specific events.** It does not impair memory of learned skills, language, or general factual information.
   5. The **patient seems unconcerned** about the memory loss.

PATIENT PROFILE

A man is involved in a car accident. He is not injured, but he cannot recall the details of the accident or what he was doing earlier that morning.

B. Dissociative fugue
1. Dissociative fugue is an **abrupt loss of memory concerning personal identity and life experience.** It usually occurs during an **emotional conflict** or after a **traumatic experience.**
2. Patients are **confused about their identity** or **assume a new identity.**
3. Patients tend to **wander far from home** and may take up a **new residence** and a **new life.**

PROFILE

After several months of increasing marital conflict, a young woman and her husband have an argument during which he batters her severely. The woman does not lose consciousness but appears dazed. After her husband leaves the house, the woman wanders outdoors and boards a bus to a nearby town, where she begins to identify herself by a new name. After a week, she recognizes herself as the woman pictured on TV as missing from the next town and goes to the police.

C. Dissociative identity disorder
1. The patient has **two or more distinct personality states.**
2. At least two of these identities **recurrently take control** of the person's behavior.
3. The person has **evident gaps in memory** (e.g., cannot recall important personal information). Typically, her memories of segments of her life (e.g., her childhood) are "blank." Current problems with memory are also present, such as the patient discovering herself in an unfamiliar neighborhood without awareness or recall of how she came to be there.
4. The patient **may not be completely aware** of the alternate identities. In fact, memory lapses signal a "switch" from one personality state to another, when these personalities (or "al-

PROFILE

A young woman named Silvia with an expressionless affect seeks treatment for depression. She complains of "forgetfulness" and "sleeping a lot." She also complains of hearing voices that "whisper mean things." Suddenly, she becomes much more animated, begins to smile and giggle, and says that she thinks Silvia is "boring" and "can't remember much." She now says that her name is Lucy and that she knows Silvia as well as Beth, who is "the tough one." Beth comes out when Silvia or Lucy is frightened. Lucy says that she gets along better with people than the others do and also has more memories of when Silvia was "touched" by her father.

ters") are unaware of each other. Sometimes these switches lead to the temporary loss of an acquired skill—such as the ability to drive a car—but the skill will be "recalled" once the alter with that memory returns to take control.

HOT

KEY

Ninety percent of patients with dissociative identity disorder were sexually abused as children.

III CAUSES

A. Essentially, dissociation is caused by **psychological trauma** that **overwhelms** the patient's **coping mechanisms.** Dissociation is an unconscious coping mechanism that suppresses memories of trauma and even intense feelings of anger or sadness. Although these traumatic memories and feelings are still present, the patient unconsciously compartmentalizes them so that she can function. The result is amnesia about certain events and many aspects of the self.

B. Dissociation is more common in people who are **easily hypnotized.** It is vital to remember that these processes are **not conscious fabrications.**

C. In its most extreme forms, dissociation fosters the development of a **new identity** and complete **abandonment of the old identity.**

    1. In dissociative fugue or dissociative identity disorder, the patient escapes memories of traumatic experiences by assuming a new identity.

    2. When **trauma is recurrent** (e.g., repeated sexual abuse), **more episodes of dissociation** occur and more identities may be created.

    3. Each alternate identity allows the patient to carry out an **important psychological function.** For example, patients with dissociative identity disorder often have an alter who "protects" the patient by being physically or mentally tough, perhaps even assuming a male identity in a female patient. Other alters may "come out" only at work or at school or when socializing. Sometimes an alter enacts the role of the abused victim (e.g., engaging in prostitution or in sexually or physically abusive relationships) or the abuser (e.g., abuses his own children).

IV APPROACH TO THE PATIENT

A. Patients who have **difficulty remembering their past** or who seem **confused about their identity** should be evaluated for a dissociative disorder.

   1. Because of their memory impairment, these patients may
   not be able to tell you much about the precipitating trauma.
   Usually, these memories are recovered only during **hypnosis**
   or while the patient is in a **medication-induced trance state**
   [e.g., amobarbital (Amytal) interview; see VI A 2 a].
   2. As much information as possible should be elicited from
   these patients, especially their **recent whereabouts** and any
   physical symptoms. All patients who have memory deficits
   should undergo an appropriate **medical evaluation** to rule
   out head trauma or other injury.
B. Patients who have dissociative identity disorder are often **unaware** of their psychological fragmentation, or they may **try to
hide** it. Initially, they often appear to have no mental illness or
may complain of mood disturbance (e.g., depression). The diagnosis may not be evident unless a shift in alters occurs during
the interview.
C. The following questions are useful in screening a patient for dissociative symptoms:
   1. Has the patient noticed episodes of "lost" time?
   2. Has the patient ever suddenly found himself somewhere,
   with no idea how he got there?
   3. Has the patient ever been recognized by people who were
   strangers to him?
   4. Has the patient discovered personal possessions in his home
   that he does not remember acquiring (e.g., clothing that is
   very different from his own)?

V DIFFERENTIAL DIAGNOSIS

A. Medical conditions. Amnesia may occur in patients who have
medical conditions that interfere with memory formation (anterograde amnesia) or recall (retrograde amnesia).
   1. Head trauma. Physical signs are usually evident. A head
   computed tomography (CT) scan or magnetic resonance
   imaging (MRI) scan should be considered.
   2. Epilepsy. A history of seizures may be evident. An electroencephalogram (EEG) may be necessary.
   3. Vascular disease. Elderly patients who have transient ischemic
   attacks (TIAs) of the areas of the brain that control memory
   formation may have transient global amnesia. It is important
   to look for a history of hypertension or coronary artery disease
   as well as focal neurologic signs of cerebrovascular disease.
   4. Encephalopathy. Acute, toxic disturbances in cerebral function are often identified by accompanying delirium and gross
   cognitive changes (e.g., inattention, fluctuating levels of
   alertness, difficulty with language). In these patients, amnesia is usually permanent.

5. **Dementia.** Patients with dementia usually have a history of chronic, progressive memory loss. In vascular dementia, however, abrupt loss of memory may follow other cognitive problems and neurologic deficits.

B. **Schizophrenia**
   1. Dissociative identity disorder may be mistaken for schizophrenia because, superficially, the patient's **account of symptoms or clinical presentation may appear psychotic.** Patients may report hearing voices (i.e., an awareness of other, alternate identities that "voice" the patient's unacceptable thoughts or feelings). Often these voices are poorly defined, but they may give specific commands (e.g., to hurt oneself).
   2. In dissociative identity disorder (but not in schizophrenia), the voices may be associated with tension-type headaches, often when the patient is under stress and several alternate identities are trying to be "out" at once.
   3. Sudden shifts between alternate identities may make the patient's behavior seem bizarre, and the patient's amnestic periods may be mistaken for poor reality testing or disorganization. To distinguish between these disorders, use the screening questions listed earlier, and explore the patient's report of any auditory hallucinations.

VI TREATMENT

A. **Dissociative amnesia and dissociative fugue**
   1. **Therapy.** The clinician may begin with supportive therapy while encouraging free association. This free association may help the patient to recover dissociated memories.
   2. **Hypnosis and medication-induced trance states.** The therapist often must rely on hypnosis or medication-induced trance states to allow repressed memories to surface.
      a. Sometimes a trance state is induced by slow intravenous infusion of **amobarbital** (Amytal). The infusion is continued until the patient begins to speak spontaneously and explore the events that led to the episode of amnesia. This procedure requires constant monitoring to avoid oversedation and respiratory depression.
      b. During hypnosis or a medication-induced trance, the clinician suggests that the patient will later consciously retain the memories, but that they will be less disturbing.
      c. After this initial intervention, further treatment is usually necessary to help the patient deal with the trauma or inner conflicts that led to the dissociative episode.

B. **Dissociative identity disorder**
   1. **Extended psychotherapy** is the primary tool used to treat these patients. The goal of therapy is to help the patient

process traumatic memories and thereby **reduce the need for defensive dissociation.**

2. These patients have very fragile coping mechanisms, so **intensive support** must be offered to ensure patient safety (e.g., behavioral contracts to refrain from suicidal behavior).

3. Because many of these patients are easily hypnotized, the therapeutic process often relies heavily on **hypnotic suggestions** that promote **healthier coping skills.** For instance, the suggestion that "younger" alters be allowed "out" only when adult behavior is not essential (e.g., when not driving or supervising one's children) may be useful.

4. Initially, the therapist focuses on **developing a rapport** with the patient. Later, the therapist encourages the patient to **explore the role of the alternative personalities** and the strengths each one brings to the person's functioning. This may ultimately facilitate greater integration.

   a. The therapist may focus on improving communication among the personalities to eliminate memory lapses.

   b. If very young personalities are present, the therapist can offer therapeutic suggestions to help them to "mature."

   c. Eventually, the therapist may be able to help the patient consolidate the personalities into one unifying personality.

VII FOLLOW-UP AND REFERRAL

A. Dissociative disorders almost always warrant **extended psychotherapy** to help the patient process psychological trauma and develop healthier coping mechanisms. This treatment requires referral to clinicians who are comfortable and skilled at handling these disorders.

B. **Medications** may be needed to treat comorbid anxiety or mood symptoms.

C. Because **substance abuse** is often present, referral for substance abuse treatment may be necessary.

References

Coons PM: Psychogenic or dissociative fugue: A clinical investigation of five cases. *Psychol Rep* 84(3):881–886, 1999.

Coons PM: The dissociative disorders: Rarely considered and underdiagnosed. *Psychiatr Clin North Am* 21(3):637–648, 1998.

Kluft RP: An overview of the psychotherapy of dissociative identity disorder. *Am J Psychother* 53(3):289–319, 1999.

PART VIII

PERSONALITY DISORDERS

23. Personality Disorders

I INTRODUCTION

A. Foundation of personality. The character traits that make up personality arise early in development. Although normal personality development continues throughout life, by puberty these character traits are **stable, enduring aspects** of a person's style of interaction.

1. A **healthy personality** is one that enables a person to adapt to stressful life situations.

2. A **personality disorder** is coded on Axis II, and according to DSM-IV, is a set of **inflexible, maladaptive** character traits that lead to **functional impairment** or cause **significant subjective distress** to the patient, in the absence of any mental state (Axis I) illness. The functional impairment arises in at least two of the following areas: cognition, affectivity, interpersonal relationships, or impulse control.

> **HOT** **KEY**
>
> Not all annoying personality traits are symptoms of a personality disorder.

B. Ineffective coping skills. People with personality disorders are easy to identify because they typically have significant **trouble with relationships, employment,** or the **law.** Because personality traits are so ingrained, it is difficult to help people with personality disorders to develop healthier coping styles.

II CLINICAL MANIFESTATIONS

A. Lack of awareness. People with personality disorders are often unaware of their inability to get along with others and function normally (e.g., hold down a job). Instead, they tend to **blame**

other people for their problems. When they experience stress in relationships or jobs, they have difficulty functioning. For instance, the temporary absence of a therapist or a significant other on vacation may provoke an overwhelming fear that the person will never return or that the person no longer cares for the patient, which may prompt desperate acts to relieve this pain (e.g., suicidal behavior).

HOT KEY

People with personality disorders tend to respond in ways that are stereotypical, rather than tailored to the situation at hand. This inflexibility leads to vicious cycles of consequences (e.g., loss of a friend when the patient becomes too intrusive or demanding) that beget behavior (e.g., frantic efforts to avoid abandonment) that begets consequences, and so on.

B. Stress. Patients who have personality disorders **cannot cope adequately with stress.** Therefore, particularly stressful situations may prompt clinically significant depressive, anxious, or even psychotic symptoms. Anxiety-prone patients (e.g., those with borderline personality disorder) may resort to **substance abuse** in an effort to cope with their feelings.

C. Normal, abnormal, and pathological traits. The current classification system for personality disorders assumes that abnormal character traits can be readily distinguished from "normal" personality traits and that the symptoms of these personality disorders are distinct from those of Axis I (i.e., mental state) disorders.

D. Classification system. Personality disorders are grouped into the following **"clusters"** according to symptom type:

1. Cluster A: "The odd ones"

PATIENT PROFILE

Paranoid Personality Disorder: The patient is a 56-year-old twice-divorced man who is in couples treatment with his third wife. The patient is angry at his wife because he believes she has had an affair with his best friend. His wife is hurt and confused, and she describes a recent encounter with his friend in which the friend innocently laid his hand on her arm during a discussion the three of them were having. This act apparently signaled treachery to the patient, leading to a desire for divorce. The patient and his wife both describe him "the jealous type," and in fact his two prior divorces occurred after similar allegations of infidelity. The patient also has great difficulty accepting criticism from co-workers and has lost or changed jobs frequently in his life due to these conflicts.

a. **Paranoid personality disorder.** People with paranoid personality disorder are suspicious of others but are not psychotic. They read hidden meanings into benign remarks or events, bear grudges, react angrily to perceived attacks, and continually question the loyalty of companions and friends.

b. **Schizoid personality disorder.** People with schizoid personality disorder are detached from social relationships (i.e., a "loner"). They appear indifferent to others' opinions, derive little pleasure from activities, and show little emotion.

PROFILE

Schizoid Personality Disorder: The patient is a 34-year-old single man whose parents bring him for evaluation because "he has no friends." The patient has always been a "loner" and never dated. He works as a computer technician, does his job, and has few, if any, outside interests. He has been resistant to leaving home, despite an evident lack of affection on his part toward his parents. The patient himself has no complaints and appears indifferent to the interviewer.

c. **Schizotypal personality disorder.** People with schizotypal personality disorder have an inappropriate affect and show pervasive social deficits (e.g., odd, almost psychotic beliefs and behaviors). They cannot develop intimate relationships because they are excessively anxious and suspicious of others.

PROFILE

Schizotypal Personality Disorder: The patient is a 29-year-old woman who sought counseling after she felt a co-worker was stealing her ideas for projects through psychic means. During an interview with a counselor, she said that the influence of this co-worker had been making her depressed and that she had sought to protect herself from this by channeling her "commotion," a process that the interviewer was unable to understand despite repeated attempts to clarify this with her. She is dressed somewhat shabbily, but with many rings on all her fingers that are somehow meaningful to this psychic protective mechanism. The patient giggles slightly while presenting her concerns, despite her complaint of feeling depressed, saying she'd really like to get to socialize with her co-workers, but they make her feel too anxious.

2. **Cluster B: "The dramatic ones"**
   a. **Borderline personality disorder.** People with borderline personality disorder have an unstable self-image. They

are emotionally volatile, have chronic feelings of empti-
ness, and fear abandonment. These patients have intense,
often inappropriate anger, and may have recurrent
thoughts of suicide. They are also impulsive and may intentionally injure themselves. They often form unstable,
intense relationships in which they either idealize or de-
value the other person.

Borderline Personality Disorder: This 24-year-old single
woman who works as a bartender entered treatment after a
recent visit to the emergency department when she cut her
wrists superficially with a knife. She has had three prior brief
hospitalizations for overdoses on medications or for cutting
herself. This last time she says she felt hopeless because her
boyfriend broke up with her, and she hoped she would "just
get his attention." She tends to binge drink and abuses other
drugs occasionally. She has a history of very intense brief relationships, mostly with men who abuse her physically. She
wonders, though, if she may also be lesbian because she finds
herself also attracted to two of her girlfriends, and she relates
this to "always looking to replace the mother who left me."

b. Histrionic personality disorder. People with histrionic
personality disorder seek attention through emotive, se-
ductive, or provocative behavior. They are shallow and
suggestible and are uncomfortable when they are not the
center of attention.

Histrionic Personality Disorder: This 44-year-old well-
dressed man is in group therapy because of his failure to
find a long-term relationship. He says, "women always call
me a Don Juan," and quickly tries to dominate the group
discussion with his dating exploits. He begins to flirt with female group members and flatters the group leader. When
pressed, however, for details about his feelings regarding
sharing in the group, he remains superficial and vague.

c. Narcissistic personality disorder. People with narcissistic
personality disorder believe that they are special but are
unconsciously quite insecure about themselves. They
have a great need for admiration and may exhibit a sense
of entitlement. They often engage in grandiose behaviors
or fantasies (e.g., unlimited success, ideal love). They cannot empathize with others.

Narcissistic Personality Disorder: This 50-year-old woman has been hospitalized because of overwhelming depression and anxiety. When initially approached by the medical student for an interview, she exclaims: "You're not a real doctor! How can I be expected to waste my time with a peon like you!" The patient continues to denigrate the student, who fearlessly persists, and eventually the patient admits she came in because she "just needs time to get my life together." It seems she has gone from doctor to doctor in search of a cure but rejects their help almost immediately as being "inadequate." Meanwhile, her private life is increasingly isolated as she has alienated all her friends and family, can't identify a job "worthy of my talents," and so is now facing bankruptcy.

d. **Antisocial personality disorder.** People with antisocial personality disorder disregard the rights and feelings of others. They are deceitful, impulsive, and aggressive and often engage in criminal behavior.

Antisocial Personality Disorder: The patient is a 25-year-old man, referred by the court for substance abuse evaluation. He has a history of multiple arrests for theft and gives accounts, almost with relish, of being truant at school so he could develop a counterfeit money-making scheme and of stealing cars for joyrides. He deals drugs at the local middle school through his second son, the only one of his five children he is in contact with (each born to a different girlfriend). He begins subtly asking the interviewer about disability because, he states, "serious" substance abusers, such as himself, need "all the help they can get."

3. **Cluster C: "The anxious ones"**
   a. **Obsessive–compulsive personality disorder.** People with obsessive–compulsive personality disorder are preoccupied with order and rules. They are perfectionistic, rigid, overly conscientious, and miserly and tend to hoard objects. This personality disorder is distinct from obsessive–compulsive disorder (OCD) (see Chapter 21), in which obsessive thoughts generate compulsive rituals. People with obsessive–compulsive personality disorder do not generally have such compulsions.
   b. **Dependent personality disorder.** People with dependent personality disorder fear the disapproval of others. They

PATIENT PROFILE

Obsessive–Compulsive Personality Disorder: A 32-year-old female attorney presents complaining of a "learning disability" that is interfering with her job. Her co-workers in the firm have become frustrated that she is unable to complete assignments on time. The patient describes feeling uncomfortable handing in assignments until "every last detail is taken care of" and so never really finishes. She denies any intrusive thoughts, or a feeling that her actions are repetitive, but does admit that she tends to organize, sort, and rearrange things to the detriment of getting more important work done. She loves to work, so much so that she tends to ignore social relationships and outside activities. She dates occasionally and had one serious relationship. Her boyfriend became frustrated, however, that she wasn't spontaneous and that she tended to be overly rigid in trying to set up "rules of conduct" for them to live by.

exhibit submissive, clinging behavior, have difficulty making everyday decisions, and rely excessively on others for emotional support.

PATIENT PROFILE

Dependent Personality Disorder: This anxious-appearing 42-year-old man is brought to the psychiatrist's office by his mother for evaluation saying, "I don't understand. He's never going to get married!" The patient himself says he thinks he's been a failure all his life and cannot imagine living on his own. He has had a few dates, but cut the relationships off, usually because he was sure his parents would disapprove of the women he chose. His mother interjects, "But we never even heard about them!" The patient chose his present job as a dental hygienist, which he dislikes, because his mother wanted him to be a dentist, but he was too afraid to leave home to attend dental school.

PATIENT PROFILE

Avoidant Personality Disorder: This 41-year-old shy-appearing woman states that she is very sad because she hasn't ever married and now will never have children. She lives alone and has only two aquaintances whom she met at her job as a clerical worker in a business nearby. She calls them "friends" but rarely has met with them socially outside of work, out of fear that they wouldn't like her if they "knew the real me." Similar anxiety prevents her from even engaging men in conversation. She avoids eye contact with the medical student during the interview and blushes several times before she admits that her one and only date in high school failed after she refused a kiss goodnight.

   c. **Avoidant personality disorder.** People with avoidant personality disorder are socially inhibited and fear being disliked or criticized. They desire relationships and feel attachment to others, but their relationships are unsatisfactory because they are dominated by feelings of inadequacy and shame.

III CAUSES

A. Personality development. Many factors probably affect the development of personality.

   1. **Genetic factors** are responsible for temperament, which is apparent even in infancy.

   2. As the child matures, **early relationships** (before 5 years of age) have a tremendous influence on the emergence of distinct personality styles.

   3. Some personality disorders seem to arise in response to **pathological parenting.** If a child does not develop a healthy sense of self, problematic behaviors and coping strategies can arise. For example, people who experience significant emotional neglect or abuse during the early years are prone to identity disturbances and may struggle with a constant fear of abandonment.

B. Alternative clustering system. Recent research has led to the creation of a different clustering system that takes into account the pathology, its etiology, and therapeutic considerations. The three clusters are as follows:

   1. **"Spectrum" personality disorders** are linked to, or on a spectrum with, their comparable **Axis I disorders.**

      a. **Paranoid personality disorder** is linked to **delusional disorder** and **schizophrenia.**

      b. **Schizotypal personality disorder** is common in relatives of people with **schizophrenia.**

   2. **"Self" personality disorders** occur in people who have **diffuse or fragile identities** as a result of abnormal development, typically due to abuse or neglect during early childhood.

      a. **Borderline personality disorder** is clearly associated with the constant threat of **emotional abandonment** in childhood.

      b. **Antisocial personality disorder** occurs most often in families that encourage **aggression** and do not provide **positive reinforcement** or set **limits. Genetic factors** may also be involved.

      c. **Schizoid personality disorder** may be related to **genetic influence** or to grossly **inadequate** or **neglectful parenting.**

   3. **"Trait" personality disorders** occur when normal personality traits are **exaggerated.**

      a. **Avoidant personality disorder** may be caused by an exaggerated **desire for acceptance.**

    b. Obsessive–compulsive personality disorder may be caused by an exaggerated attempt to be perfect to please controlling, rigid parents. A biologic component is also evident.

    c. Histrionic personality disorder appears to be inherited and is associated with conflict over attachment to parents.

    d. Dependent personality disorder also appears to be inherited and can occur when parents do not tolerate aggression or autonomy in the child.

    e. Narcissistic personality disorder can occur in people whose parents are strongly disapproving and show little empathy. Because of resultant feelings of inferiority, the person continually devalues or demeans others as a way of not being hurt first. In other words, in narcissistic personality disorder, "the best defense is a good offense."

IV ▌ APPROACH TO THE PATIENT

A. Inherent difficulty with relationships. People with personality disorders have trouble with relationships. They bring this tendency to the physician–patient relationship as well.

> **HOT** **KEY** During the initial patient interview, the clinician's response to the patient's style is usually significant. Patients with personality disorders can really "push your buttons"!

B. Chronic problem. Although patients with personality disorders may be in crisis at the time of evaluation, their difficulties are chronic.

C. Underlying conditions. It is important to assess the patient carefully for the presence of treatable Axis I symptoms that may be fueling the current situation.

D. Specific concerns

    1. Patients with **borderline** and **narcissistic personality disorders** are especially likely to idealize or devalue physicians and other staff.

    2. Patients with **antisocial personality disorder** may attempt to manipulate the physician to achieve a desired goal (e.g., food, medication, safe haven).

E. Avoiding manipulation. It is best to refrain from reacting to the patient's attempts to manipulate the situation and instead to help these patients adjust their expectations by providing some reality checks. For these patients, the best approach is to provide support (empathize), clarify the issues at hand, and outline realistic goals.

V TREATMENT

A. Therapy. Successful treatment often includes **psychotherapy** (ranging from cognitive–behavioral to psychodynamic techniques), **interventions for substance abuse,** and **family** or **group psychotherapy.**

B. Medications. Some people benefit from medication to decrease **impulsive behavior** and treat comorbid **mood or anxiety disorders.**

C. If a patient exhibits **dangerous behavior,** clear **limit-setting** is essential. **Hospitalization,** even briefly, also may be appropriate.

VI FOLLOW-UP AND REFERRAL

A. Patients who have personality disorders often seek treatment for **specific problems.** However, they may not realize that they perpetuate their own problems through their behavior.

HOT

KEY

The patient with a personality disorder requires long-term management.

B. These patients require appropriate **crisis intervention,** followed by **referral** to a mental health practitioner who is comfortable addressing these disorders.

C. Referral for **substance abuse treatment** also may be necessary.

References

Marlowe M, Sugarman P: ABC of mental health. Disorders of personality. *BMJ* 315(7101):176–179, 1997.

Perry JC, Banon E, Ianni F: Effectiveness of psychotherapy for personality disorders. *Am J Psychiatry* 156(9):1312–1321, 1999.

Silk KR: Borderline personality disorder. Overview of biologic factors. *Psychiatr Clin North Am* 23(1):61–75, 2000.

PART IX

Consultation–Liaison Issues

24. Capacity Assessment

◼ Introduction

A. **Consultation–liaison psychiatry** is the term given to duties performed by the psychiatric consultant in the medical hospital. The focus is on areas in which there is an interface between a patient's medical and psychiatric conditions. The liaison aspect focuses upon helping staff to understand the psychiatric and psychosocial issues facing their patients.

B. **Capacity assessment,** described in this chapter, **is the evaluation of a patient's ability to understand and make decisions about his medical condition.**

C. **Physicians make judgments** about a patient's capacity regarding his medical care.

1. The assessment of a patient's decision-making capacity can be carried out by any physician; however, it is frequently the consultation–liaison psychiatrist who is called upon to do so by the referring physician.

2. The assessment includes evaluating whether a patient has the capacity to participate in medical decision making or to give consent to treatment.

3. The assessment is usually sought when a patient does not follow treatment recommendations or wishes to leave the hospital against medical advice.

D. **Competency** (as compared to capacity) is a **legal concept** concerning a person's ability to make legal decisions and is determined by the court. A physician cannot declare a patient to be incompetent. **Financial management** and **guardianship** are examples of situations in which competency determinations are made.

E. **Patients who suffer from psychiatric illness** do not automatically lose decision-making capacity. The physician must consider each individual patient's particular deficits and abilities. Also, a patient's ability to participate in medical decision making may fluctuate with progression or improvement of the illness; therefore, frequent reassessment is necessary.

HOT Capacity is not an all-or-nothing phenomenon. The first question to the referring doctor should be "capacity for what?" For example, a patient may not have capacity to participate in discharge planning but may have capacity to consent to a pro-
KEY cedure.

II APPROACH TO THE PATIENT

A. Four criteria must be considered in capacity assessment, which can be easily remembered with the following mnemonic:

Four Criteria for Capacity Assessment ("**C**apacity **F**or **C**onsultation **L**iaison")

Choice
Facts
Consequences
Logic

1. **Choice: Can the patient communicate and sustain a choice** for a reasonable period? If the patient refuses to speak or is unwilling to express a preference, he lacks capacity. This is at times seen if a patient is delirious or catatonic or has severe character pathology.
2. **Facts: Does the patient understand the relevant facts** about her condition? Has the physician provided the patient with a clear explanation of the procedure or situation at hand? Were the **risks and benefits** clearly stated and can the patient repeat them? A patient with low intelligence quotient (IQ), severe dementia, or poor attention span may not be able to fulfill this criterion.
3. **Consequences: Can the patient appreciate and understand consequences?** Can he clearly state the pros and cons of his decision? Does the patient understand that his welfare is at stake? A patient who demonstrates extreme denial may not meet this criterion.
4. **Logic: Can the patient process information rationally?** Does the patient reason logically? The examiner must pay attention to the process of decision making and not simply the outcome. Patients who are suffering from delusions or auditory hallucinations may fail this criterion.

B. If the physician determines that a patient lacks decision-making capacity, the next of kin will be asked to consent for the patient. If no health care proxy is in place, the spouse will be consulted, then children, siblings, and significant others. If the patient has no family or significant other, the hospital will petition the court to appoint a surrogate decision maker.

References
*Appelbaum PS, Grisso T: Assessing patient's capacities to consent to treatment. *N Engl J Med* 319:1635–1638, 1988.
Etchells E, Darzins P, Silberfeld M, et al: Assessment of patient capacity to consent to treatment. *J Gen Intern Med* 14(1):27–34, 1999.
Etchells E, Sharpe G, Elliott C, Singer PA: Bioethics for clinicians: Capacity. *CMAJ* 155(6):657–661, 1996.

*Classic reference

25. Delirium

I INTRODUCTION

A. **Delirium** is the most frequent reason for a psychiatric consultation in the medical setting.

B. Delirium consists of:
1. A **change in mental status** characterized by:
   a. **Disturbance in consciousness**—the patient is unable to focus and sustain attention.
   b. **Changes in cognition**—the patient may have memory deficits, perceptual disturbances, and orientation or language abnormalities.
   c. **Acute onset**—onset occurs in hours to days, with fluctuation in mental status.
2. The change in mental status is **directly related to a general medical condition, substance intoxication or withdrawal,** or **multiple etiologies.**

HOT KEY

Delirium should not be confused with dementia, which represents chronic, irreversible cognitive deterioration. Delirium is an acute, fluctuating, and largely reversible process.

C. **Causes. The etiology of delirium is almost always medical as opposed to psychiatric.** The psychiatrist is generally called because of behavioral manifestations (e.g., the patient is pulling out intravenous lines) or because the physician has difficulty ascertaining the patient's mental status.

D. **Prevalence and prognosis.** Delirium occurs in up to 20% of hospitalized patients and causes great morbidity. If the underlying cause can be effectively treated, delirium is almost always reversible.

E. **Risk factors** for developing delirium include:
1. **Young or old age** (children and the elderly)
2. **Structural brain abnormalities** (e.g., related to stroke, dementia, or epilepsy)
3. **Recent major surgery** (especially hip and cardiac surgery)
4. **Polypharmacy**
5. Infection with the human immunodeficiency virus **(HIV)**—15% of patients with advanced HIV disease develop HIV-1-associated dementia (HAD) (see Chapter 28 II).

HOT **KEY**

Delirium represents acute brain dysfunction. It is always a medical emergency.

II CLINICAL MANIFESTATIONS

A. Frequently there is a **prodromal phase** in which the patient is restless, anxious, and irritable, with a reversal in the sleep cycle (sedation during the day, wakefulness at night).

B. **Changes in consciousness**
1. Lucid intervals fluctuate with periods of confusion or agitation.
2. The patient is oriented to person but not to time or place.
3. Paranoid or persecutory delusions are often present.

C. **Changes in cognition**
1. Memory for recent events is impaired.
2. The patient has trouble maintaining focus and attention.
3. Thought disturbances such as disorganization, derailment, and perseveration are common.

D. **Other manifestations**
1. **Perceptual disturbances,** such as illusions or visual, tactile, or auditory hallucinations, may occur.
2. **Psychomotor abnormalities** range from severe hyperactivity (e.g., in alcohol withdrawal) to hypoactivity (e.g., in elderly patients with urinary tract infections).
3. A patient's **affect** is frequently altered and labile.

III DIFFERENTIAL DIAGNOSIS. The psychiatric consultant

Etiology of Delirium ("WHHHHIMP")

Withdrawal (usually from alcohol or benzodiazepines) or **W**ernicke's encephalopathy
Hypoxemia or **H**ypercapnia
Hypertension
Hypoglycemia
Hypoperfusion of the brain
Infection or **I**ntracranial bleed
Meningitis or **M**etabolic derangement (liver, kidney, thyroid, parathyroid, adrenal, acid-base)
Poisons (illicit drugs) or medications
(Modified from Rundell JR, Wise MC: *Textbook of Consultation Liaison Psychiatry.* Washington, DC, American Psychiatric Press, 1996.)

should help the medical team to determine the particular etiology of the patient's delirium. The mnemonic "WHHHHIMP" can guide the investigation.

IV APPROACH TO THE PATIENT

A. The patient must be assessed at least every day and often more frequently. A diagnosis of delirium can be missed if the patient is examined only during a lucid interval.

   1. Notes pertaining to **sleep** should be reviewed.

   2. In hospitalized patients, **very recent medications** (including those given as needed) should be noted. Even a small amount of opioids or benzodiazepines in the elderly can lead to delirium.

HOT KEY It is important to get collateral history from family, nursing staff, or emergency department notes, and medication and anesthesia records.

   3. A careful **mental status examination** should be done, paying particular attention to orientation, memory, language, perceptual disturbances, and psychomotor activity.

   4. The patient should be asked to write a sentence, draw a clock, or do the Trail Making Test (a test that requires connecting randomly placed numbers or connecting letters of the alphabet with numbers). Patients with delirium will have difficulties with these tasks.

   5. A careful **neurologic examination** should be performed, focusing on asterixis (indicates hepatic or uremic encephalopathy), myoclonus [indicates lithium or meperidine (Demerol) toxicity], nystagmus [indicates phenytoin (Dilantin) or phencyclidine (PCP) toxicity] and oculomotor palsy (indicates sixth nerve palsy of Wernicke's encephalopathy).

B. Basic work-up usually includes:

   1. Complete blood cell (CBC) count

   2. Chemistry panel

   3. Liver and thyroid studies

   4. Urine culture and sensitivity test and urine toxicology test

   5. Chest radiograph

   6. Head computed tomography (CT) or magnetic resonance imaging (MRI)

   7. Consider lumbar puncture (LP) if there are signs of meningitis

   8. Consider electroencephalogram (EEG) (may show generalized slowing of background rhythm)

   9. Consider arterial blood gas (ABG)

V TREATMENT

A. General management

1. **The underlying cause** should be treated; however, the etiologies of the delirium may not always be identified.
2. The patient must be kept **safe.**

B. Medications

1. **Haloperidol** (Haldol) may be used parenterally, intramuscularly, or by mouth (e.g., 1–2 mg every 1–2 hours) until the patient is calm. **Lorazepam** (Ativan) (e.g., 1–2 mg every 1–2 hours) may be used in conjunction with haloperidol if the patient is severely agitated.
2. **Anticholinergic drugs,** such as diphenhydramine (Benadryl) or benztropine (Cogentin), **should be avoided.**

C. Environmental manipulation.
The patient should be moved closer to the nursing station. One-to-one observation should be assigned. Family members should be asked to bring calendars or objects from home to help with orientation.

D. Reassurance and education of the family.
The physician should reassure and educate the family members, who are often devastated to see the patient's agitation, confusion, and change in personality.

References

Cole MG, Primeau F, McCusker J: Effectiveness of interventions to prevent delirium in hospitalized patients: A systematic review. *CMAJ* 155(9):1263–1268, 1996.

Jacobson S, Schreibman B: Behavioral and pharmacologic treatment of delirium. *Am Fam Physician* 56(8):2005–2012, 1997.

Trzepacz PT: Delirium: Advances in diagnosis, pathophysiology and treatment. *Psychiatr Clin North Am* 19(3):429–448, 1996.

26. Death and Grief

I INTRODUCTION

A. Medical training focuses on the diagnosis and cure of the patient. When confronted with the dying patient, there is a tendency to feel helpless, anxious, and uncomfortable. Dealing with the dying patient gives rise to feelings about one's own mortality, which may lead the clinician to avoid the patient. However, these patients have a right to care, and working with a terminally ill patient or patient's family can be a very gratifying process.

B. When patients receive news of a terminal illness, psychological adaptation occurs as delineated in the following five stages described by Kübler-Ross.

Kübler-Ross's Five Stages of Grief ("DABDA")

Denial
Anger
Bargaining
Depression
Acceptance

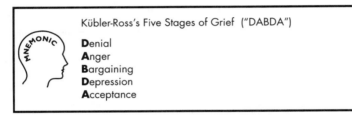

HOT KEY

Not all patients go through all of these stages, which may be experienced in any order.

Patients experience a wide range of emotions and may have many fears including abandonment, disfigurement, loss of autonomy, and pain. In most cases a psychiatric consultation is not requested, unless the patient experiences anxiety, depression, intractable pain, delirium, or severe denial.

II CLINICAL MANIFESTATIONS SPECIFIC TO THE DYING PATIENT

A. Anxiety

1. **Adjustment disorder with anxious mood** may be seen as a reaction to the impending loss of life and separation from loved ones.

    2. Disease and treatment-related anxiety

      a. Patients with sepsis, fever, metabolic abnormalities (e.g., acidosis, hypoxemia), pulmonary embolism, or myocardial infarction can present with anxiety.

      b. Anxiety may be induced by medications such as bronchodilators, antiemetics [i.e., prochlorperazine (Compazine)], glucocorticoids, or thyroid supplements.

      c. Patients withdrawing from alcohol, benzodiazepines, or opioids usually present with prominent anxiety.

    3. Preexisting anxiety disorders. In the face of terminal illness, prior anxiety disorders may reemerge. For example, breathing difficulty may precipitate panic disorder, or painful medical procedures may precipitate phobias or posttraumatic stress disorder (PTSD).

B. Depression

    1. Depression may be a prominent symptom in **medical illnesses** such as central nervous system (CNS) lymphoma, pancreatic cancer, lung cancer, or paraneoplastic syndromes.

    2. Depression is more common in **advanced disease.**

    3. Depression may be **secondary to medications** such as glucocorticoids and chemotherapy agents (e.g., vincristine, vinblastine, asparaginase, and intrathecal methotrexate).

III APPROACH TO THE PATIENT AND TREATMENT

A. Treatment for preexisting anxiety disorders—benzodiazepines, antipsychotics

B. Treatment for depression—antidepressants, psychostimulants

C. Treatment for pain—patients should receive standing pain medication rather than medication "as needed."

    1. Dosing intervals should be short (i.e., every 3–4 hours).

    2. If possible, opioids should be changed to long-acting forms.

    3. Tricyclic antidepressants or psychostimulants can augment analgesic action.

D. Emotional care. The physician should:

    1. Listen to the patient and provide consistent contact.

    2. Get to know the patient's family and provide support.

    3. Sit down next to the patient when delivering bad news and be concise. **The physician needs to be truthful but to give the patient hope and confidence that she will not be abandoned.**

    4. Collaborate with pastoral care or social work staff.

E. Management of bereavement

    1. Mourning often occurs in three phases:

      a. Preoccupation with the lost person. Survivors may hold conversations with the departed or report sensing their presence.

      b. Disorganization and despair

    c. Reorganization and restoration of normal functioning
2. The length of bereavement varies among individuals and among cultures.
3. Major depressive disorder is usually not diagnosed in the bereaved unless the symptoms of despair and depression are severe and prolonged (i.e., occur for more than 6 months). Symptoms that may be present in depression but not in normal grief include suicidality, preoccupation with worthlessness, guilt, marked psychomotor retardation, and hallucinations unrelated to the deceased.

References

*Bowlby J: Process of mourning. *Int J Psychoanal* 43:317–340, 1961.

Krigger KW, McNelly JD, Lippmann SB: Dying, death, and grief. Helping patients and their families through the process. *Postgrad Med* 101(3):263–270, 1997.

Krohn B: When death is near: Helping families cope. *Geriatric Nursing* 19(5):276–278, 1998.

*Kübler-Ross E: *On Death and Dying.* New York, Macmillan, 1969.

Stroebe M, van Son M, Stroebe W, et al: On the classification and diagnosis of pathological grief. *Clin Psychol Rev* 20(1):57–75, 2000.

*Classic reference

27. Unexplained Somatic Symptoms and Somatoform Disorders

....

I INTRODUCTION

A. Unexplained somatic complaints. The majority of the general population frequently experience **a physical symptom for which there is no identifiable organic cause.** Common somatic complaints for which a medical evaluation is often negative include **headache, fatigue, dizziness,** and **palpitations.** If these symptoms persist despite the best effort of the treating physician, a psychiatric consultation may be requested.

B. Many patients with **psychiatric illnesses present with somatic symptoms. Other psychiatric disorders should be ruled out** before somatoform disorders are suspected.

   1. Patients with major depressive disorders often present with somatic symptoms (e.g., fatigue, aches and pains).

   2. Panic disorder (e.g., chest pain, palpitations, difficulty breathing)

   3. Generalized anxiety disorder (e.g., gastrointestinal symptoms, back pain, headache)

   4. Substance use disorders

C. In malingering and factitious disorder, symptom production is conscious. By contrast, **somatoform disorders** are a spectrum of illnesses in which symptom production is unconscious and originates from **unconscious** motives and conflicts.

II CLINICAL MANIFESTATIONS, APPROACH TO THE PATIENT, AND TREATMENT

A. Malingering

   1. A patient lies about his symptoms and symptom severity because of an **external incentive** (secondary gain). Such incentives may include avoidance of work, obtaining monetary rewards, evasion of criminal prosecution, or obtaining drugs.

   2. If the patient discusses his symptoms in a medicolegal context or does not cooperate with the diagnostic evaluation, malingering should be suspected.

   3. Often there is a marked discrepancy between objective findings and the patient's reported distress. Frequently these patients have an underlying antisocial personality disorder.

    4. When malingering is strongly suspected, the patient should usually be confronted.

B. Factitious disorder

    1. Patients with factitious disorder (sometimes known as **Munchausen syndrome**) report psychological symptoms or **inflict physical harm on themselves** in the absence of obvious external motives or incentives.

    2. There is a strong desire to remain in the **sick role,** and the patient's behavior is driven by psychopathology.

    3. Many of the patients with this disorder are women under 40 years of age who have gained medical sophistication by working in health care settings or having had a true physical illness.

    4. Borderline personality disorder or dependent, masochistic, or histrionic personality traits may be seen, but there is often no specific Axis I or II disorder (see Chapters 1 and 23).

    5. Examples of self-inflicted conditions include:

        a. Self-induced infections from injection of contaminated material

        b. Factitious fever from tampering with the thermometer

        c. Factitious hypoglycemia from ingestion of an oral anti-hyperglycemic or from insulin injections

        d. Self-inflicted dermatitides from scratching, burning, or picking of skin

        e. Factitious anemia from performing phlebotomy or self-administration of warfarin (Coumadin) with subsequent bleeding

    6. When a factitious disorder is suspected, careful evaluation of prior medical records and collateral history and performance of a room search are essential. Often the patient will not cooperate with questioning or may "flee" the hospital if she suspects discovery. When discussing the diagnosis with the patient, it is helpful to point out that no incurable disease was found, but nonetheless there is great emotional suffering, which could be alleviated by obtaining counseling.

C. Somatoform disorders. Somatoform disorders are characterized by physical symptoms for which no physical cause can be identified but which are linked to psychological conflicts.

    1. Conversion disorder

        a. Definition. The patient with conversion disorder experiences a **loss or change in sensory or motor function** in response to **temporally related** meaningful **psychological stressors.** The symptoms may help patients unconsciously deal with a psychological conflict (e.g., a draftee who develops a paralyzed arm).

      b. Clinical manifestations. Patients may report blindness or tunnel vision or demonstrate gait or coordination disturbances. They may experience paralysis, seizures, or anesthesia. These symptoms are **not voluntarily** produced. Conversion disorder is more common in women and in patients suffering from depression or anxiety. In as many as 30% of patients diagnosed with conversion disorder, however, an organic cause (e.g., multiple sclerosis) will be found in the ensuing years, explaining previous "conversion symptoms."

      c. Approach to the patient and **treatment.** Hypnosis or an interview after the administration of amobarbital sodium (an "Amytal interview") can help with the diagnosis. In these states, the symptoms typically disappear. Confrontation should be avoided. Treatment consists of reassurance that no incurable illness exists and suggestion that a recovery is likely, although it may happen slowly. These patients often gradually recover in the hospital.

2. Body dysmorphic disorder

      a. Definition. These patients are preoccupied and **obsessed** with an exaggerated or **imagined physical bodily defect** (see Chapter 21 V E).

      b. Clinical manifestations. Patients may focus on flaws of the face (i.e., length of nose, shape of chin, or wrinkles) or experience concern about breast, genitalia, or other body parts. Average onset of symptoms is before 20 years of age, with equal representation of men and women. Frequently, patients with body dysmorphic disorder will also suffer from atypical depression, social phobia, or obsessive–compulsive disorder.

      c. Approach to the patient and **treatment.** Patients may respond to a trial with a selective serotonin reuptake inhibitor. If the preoccupation is of delusional proportion, an antipsychotic such as pimozide (Orap) may be indicated.

3. Hypochondriasis

      a. Definition. The hallmark of hypochondriasis is the patient's preoccupation with the belief that he is suffering from a serious medical illness. The disturbance must last at least 6 months and not be delusional in intensity.

      b. Clinical manifestations. Despite lack of medical evidence and frequent reassurance, patients with this disorder spend a great deal of time focusing on their own health and bodies. Compulsive traits, anxiety, and depression frequently coexist. The disorder is equally represented among men and women and generally has a chronic course.

      c. Approach to the patient and **treatment.** These patients need help in coping with symptoms. Treatment consists of helping the patient to understand that no medical intervention will take away the need to feel ill. The physician should avoid unnecessary diagnostic tests and surgical interventions. Patients should have regular follow-up visits, and the physician should attempt to get to know each as a person, rather than focusing exclusively on physical concerns.

4. Pain disorder

  a. Definition. Chronic, severe pain with no medical etiology is the main feature of this disorder. Psychological factors are judged to play a role in the onset, maintenance, or exacerbation of the pain. The pain is not intentionally produced or feigned.

  b. Clinical manifestations. As many as 50% of patients with pain disorder suffer from major depression and almost all suffer from dysthymia.

  c. Approach to the patient and **treatment.** Treatment involves reassurance and support. Acute pain requires aggressive treatment to prevent development of chronic pain. Hypnosis may be of help as well.

5. Somatization disorder

  a. Definition. This is a polysymptomatic illness that usually begins before 30 years of age. According to DSM-IV, at least **four pain** symptoms, **two gastrointestinal** symptoms, **one sexual** symptom, and **one pseudoneurologic** symptom are required in order to meet diagnostic criteria.

  b. Clinical manifestations. The disorder is more common in women and in patients of lower socioeconomic groups. Psychiatric comorbidities may include depression, anxiety, and substance abuse disorders. A seven-symptom screening test developed by Othmer and DeSouza uses the mnemonic: "**S**omatization **D**isorder **B**esets **L**adies **A**nd **V**exes **P**hysicians." If two or more symptoms are present, there is a high likelihood that somatization disorder is present.

Symptoms of Somatization Disorder ("**S**omatization **D**isorder **B**esets **L**adies **A**nd **V**exes **P**hysicians")

Shortness of breath
Dysmenorrhea
Burning in sex organ
Lump in throat (difficulty swallowing)
Amnesia
Vomiting
Painful extremities
(Othmer E, DeSouza D: A screening test for somatization disorder. *Am J Psychiatry* 142:1146–1149, 1985.)

c. **Approach to the patient** and **treatment**

(1) The diagnosis is often difficult to make, and collateral information from old charts, hospital records, and history from families may help. Patients with somatization disorders are typically poor historians, providing only vague and elusive details. Complaints tend to be presented in histrionic fashion.

(2) This is a chronic disorder with a relatively poor prognosis.

HOT

KEY

It is important that one physician coordinate the medical care of patients with somatization disorder.

It is helpful for the physician to develop a supportive relationship with the patient and focus the therapy on the psychosocial issues. Diagnostic evaluation should be limited.

(3) Regular, short appointments are helpful, and a brief physical examination should be performed to assess somatic complaints.

References

Barsky A, Borus JF: Functional somatic syndromes [review]. *Ann Intern Med* 130(11):910–921, 1999.

Epstein RM, Quill TE, McWhinney IR: Somatization reconsidered: Incorporating the patient's experience of illness. *Arch Intern Med* 159(3):215–222, 1999.

McCahill ME: Somatoform and related disorders: Delivery of diagnosis as first step. *Am Fam Physician* 52(1):193–204, 1995.

28. Psychiatric Aspects of Human Immunodeficiency Virus (HIV)

▮ I ▮ INTRODUCTION

A. Human immunodeficiency virus (HIV) infection is associated with a number of neuropsychiatric disorders. These include cognitive disorders, mood disorders, and psychotic disorders.

B. In addition, HIV-infected patients may have underlying psychiatric illness or develop neuropsychiatric side effects from medication (see Table 28-1).

▮ II ▮ DEMENTIA DUE TO HIV DISEASE

A. Introduction. Dementia due to HIV disease, also referred to as HIV-1-associated dementia (HAD), involves the subcortical region of the brain. The prevalence of at least moderately severe HAD is estimated to be about 15% in patients with ad-

TABLE 28-1. Possible Neuropsychiatric Side Effects of Common Medications Used in Patients with HIV Disease

Medication	Possible Neuropsychiatric Side Effects
Acyclovir	Visual hallucinations, confusion, insomnia
Amphotericin B	Delirium
Dideoxyinosine (DDI)	Insomnia, mania
Ganciclovir	Mania, psychosis, delirium, irritability, or agitation
Interferon α	Depression
Isoniazid	Depression, agitation, hallucinations, paranoia, or impaired memory
Methotrexate	Encephalopathy (in high doses)
Steroids	Depression, psychosis, or mania
Zidovudine [azidothymidine (AZT)]	Agitation, insomnia, depression, irritability, or mania

vanced HIV disease. Although about 50% of patients with acquired immune deficiency syndrome (AIDS) have a mild neurocognitive disorder, not all of these patients develop a full dementia syndrome.

B. Clinical features. HAD is characterized by the following:

1. **Cognitive impairment**—mental slowing, impairment in short-term memory, and diminished concentration, attention, and executive functioning

2. **Motor deficits**—diminished fine-motor speed, control, coordination, and possibly, ataxia

3. **Affective and behavioral effects**—possible apathetic, depressed, or labile mood as well as social withdrawal, mutism, or psychosis

C. Diagnosis. HAD is a clinical diagnosis based on results of a comprehensive history as well as brain imaging, lumbar puncture, neuropsychological testing, and certain blood tests.

1. **Imaging.** Computed tomography (CT) and magnetic resonance imaging (MRI) may reveal cerebral atrophy and ventricular enlargement. MRI may also show increased white signal intensity, a space-occupying lesion (e.g., toxoplasmosis or lymphoma), or progressive multifocal leukoencephalopathy (PML).

2. **Laboratory tests.** The cerebrospinal fluid (CSF) may reveal nonspecific changes (e.g., a mild increase in protein and a mononuclear pleocytosis) but can be used to exclude infections (e.g., cryptococcal meningitis, toxoplasmosis, or syphilis). Useful blood tests include a complete blood cell (CBC) count, serum chemistries, vitamin B_{12} level, thyroid-stimulating hormone (TSH), and rapid plasma reagin (RPR) tests.

3. **Neuropsychological testing,** such as the Trail Making Test, Finger Tapping Test, or Grooved Pegboard Test, can aid in the diagnosis. The HIV Dementia Rating Scale is generally a more useful screening test than the Mini Mental State Examination, because the patient's mental status is rarely impaired until advanced stages of HAD.

D. Treatment

1. Zidovudine [azidothymidine (AZT)] is a nucleoside antiretroviral agent used for treatment of HAD, which is thought to work by direct inhibition of HIV replication. It readily crosses the blood-brain barrier and can improve cognitive functioning and therefore may delay the progression of HAD.

2. HAD can also be treated symptomatically using the psychostimulants dextroamphetamine or methylphenidate (5–30 mg of each, which may be divided into morning and mid-day doses). These agents can improve concentration and atten-

tion as well as dysphoria and apathy. Low doses can be effective and are generally well tolerated.

3. Neuroleptics in low doses, such as haloperidol, 0.5–5.0 mg, can effectively treat psychosis associated with HAD.

4. Psychosocial interventions including support of the patient and caretaker, behavioral management, and cognitive retraining can be an important part of comprehensive treatment.

5. Patients with advanced HAD may require placement in a supervised setting.

III DELIRIUM ASSOCIATED WITH HIV DISEASE

A. Delirium is among the most frequent neuropsychiatric complications in hospitalized patients with AIDS. It is greatly underdiagnosed.

B. Underlying HAD can predispose patients to the development of delirium. There are often multiple contributing factors including metabolic abnormalities, systemic or intracranial infection, side effects of medication, intracranial neoplasm, seizure disorder or postictal states, drug or alcohol withdrawal, hypoglycemia, hypoxia, anemia, renal or liver impairment, and other disorders.

C. Management involves identification and treatment of the underlying etiology. Neuroleptics are used for symptomatic management of agitation. Low doses of haloperidol, risperidone, or olanzapine can be effective (see Chapter 25 V).

IV MOOD DISORDERS WITH HIV DISEASE

A. **Depression**

1. **Introduction.** Major depression is a common reason for psychiatric consultation in HIV and AIDS patients. It is diagnosed in up to an estimated 15% of hospitalized patients with HIV or AIDS seen by the psychiatric consultation–liaison service.

It is essential that health care workers recognize and treat depression in HIV and AIDS patients and not consider it a normal response to HIV infection.

2. **Causes.** Depression may occur as an underlying psychiatric illness or may be related to the HIV disease or its treatment. It may occur in association with HAD, with central nervous system (CNS) infection, or with systemic HIV disease. En-

docrine and metabolic disturbances, such as adrenocortical insufficiency, thyroid disease, vitamin B_{12} deficiency, hypotestosterone states, and protein and caloric malnutrition may contribute.

3. **Clinical manifestations.** It can be difficult to interpret symptoms such as changes in sleep, appetite, or energy when assessing depression in this population; it may be more useful to assess factors such as hopelessness, anhedonia, and suicidal thoughts.

4. **Approach to the patient.** HIV-infected patients are at a significantly higher risk for suicide compared with non-HIV-infected patients in their age group; suicide risk should be carefully assessed in this population.

5. **Treatment**
   a. **Pharmacological treatment** includes selective serotonin reuptake inhibitors (SSRIs), tricyclic antidepressants, and psychostimulants (see Chapter 16). Medications should be initiated at low doses and titrated slowly.
      (1) SSRIs, such as fluoxetine, paroxetine, and sertraline, may be useful in treating major depression related to HIV.
      (2) Tricyclic antidepressants. Nortriptyline, desipramine, and imipramine may be better tolerated than amitriptyline and doxepin, both of which can lead to significant anticholinergic side effects such as sedation or confusion.
      (3) The psychostimulants dextroamphetamine and methylphenidate can improve mood, energy, appetite, ability to concentrate, and attention. Usual doses range from 5 to 30 mg. Onset of action is generally rapid, and abuse is uncommon.
   b. **Psychotherapeutic techniques** including supportive therapy, cognitive behavioral therapy, and group therapy can be useful in addressing psychosocial issues including adjustment to a diagnosis of HIV and coping with grief.

B. **Mania** (see Chapter 17 II A)
   1. An acute manic episode in an HIV-infected patient may be due to underlying bipolar disorder or may be secondary to a toxic or metabolic process, a space-occupying lesion, a CNS opportunistic infection or tumor, HAD, or side effects of medication.
   2. HAD can be associated with periods of irritability and hypomania.
   3. The evaluation of the new onset of mania in an HIV patient should include brain imaging and review of the patient's current medication. An examination of the CSF may be indicated.
   4. Lithium can be useful for the treatment of mania although anticonvulsants may prove more effective in this population.

Adjunctive treatment includes high-potency neuroleptics with close monitoring for possible emergence of extrapyramidal symptoms (EPS). Benzodiazepines may also be effective. When using valproic acid, liver function tests (LFTs), CBC counts, and coagulation factors should be monitored. Valproic acid is generally considered preferable to carbamazepine, which can suppress the white blood cells (WBCs).

V PSYCHOSIS WITH HIV DISEASE

A. The differential diagnosis of psychosis (see Chapter 9) in an HIV patient includes underlying psychiatric disorders such as schizophrenia or bipolar disorder, delirium, advanced dementia, substance use disorders, and neurologic conditions such as complex partial seizures. It may occur in the context of a CNS infection or other CNS complications of HIV or as a medication side effect.

B. Treatment involves the use of neuroleptics. Clozapine is not recommended because of potential WBC suppression and the risk of seizures. The underlying cause of the psychosis should be treated if possible.

VI ANXIETY DISORDERS WITH HIV DISEASE

A. Anxiety disorders are common in patients with HIV and AIDS.

B. Causes. There may be an underlying psychiatric disorder such as an adjustment disorder, posttraumatic stress disorder (PTSD), panic disorder, generalized anxiety disorder (GAD), or obsessive–compulsive disorder (OCD). Stressors such as the HIV diagnosis, starting antiretroviral treatment, or a declining CD4+ lymphocyte count may be precipitants. Anxiety may also result from metabolic disturbance such as anemia, hypoxia, hypoglycemia, complex partial seizures, CNS complications of HIV, systemic illness, or side effects of medication.

C. Treatment. Pharmacological treatment includes buspirone and benzodiazepines, and there may be a role for β-adrenergic blockers, antihistamines, or antidepressants in certain situations. Psychotherapy, either cognitive or behavioral, may be effective alone or in conjunction with medication.

References

Policy guideline on the recognition and management of HIV-related neuropsychiatric findings and associated impairments. *Am J Psychiatry* 155(11):1647, 1998.

Rabkin JG, Ferrando SJ, Jacobsberg LB, et al: Prevalence of axis I disorders in an AIDS cohort: A cross-sectional, controlled study. *Compr Psychiatry* 38(3):146–154, 1997.

Rabkin JG, Wagner GJ, Rabkin R: Fluoxetine treatment for depression in patients with HIV and AIDS: A randomized, placebo-controlled trial. *Am J Psychiatry* 156(1):101–107, 1999.

29. Psychiatric Disorders During Pregnancy and Postpartum

I. INTRODUCTION

A. Pregnancy. While preexisting psychiatric disorders may present a problem during pregnancy, **it is unusual for new conditions to present during this time.**

B. Postpartum period. The postpartum period, however, is **an extremely vulnerable period** for both the exacerbation of affective and psychotic disorders and the emergence of a first episode of psychiatric illness.

II. PREGNANCY.

The **diagnostic criteria for psychiatric disorders in pregnancy are the same** as those for the nonpregnant state. The approach to treatment differs.

A. Approach to the patient

> **HOT KEY**
>
> As a general principle, the lowest possible dose of medication should be used, with exposure to as few agents as possible during pregnancy.

1. For nonpsychotic illnesses such as most depressive and anxiety disorders, **nonpharmaceutical treatment modalities should be strongly considered.** These may include psychotherapy, temporary lifestyle changes, light therapy, sleep hygiene techniques, hypnosis, and hospitalization.

2. **Electroconvulsive therapy** is also a safe and viable option when performed under conditions appropriate for pregnancy.

> **HOT KEY**
>
> While the goal of treatment for a patient in the nonpregnant state is a complete resolution of symptoms, during pregnancy the goal is to reach a **tolerable level** of symptoms. It is important to remember that a "tolerable level" will be different for each individual.

B. Risks are involved with prenatal exposure to medications.

1. The risks associated with fetal exposure to medication must be weighed against the risks of untreated psychiatric illness including neglect of prenatal care, suicidality, impulsivity, and risk of treatment resistance secondary to repeated relapses.

2. **Three categories** of possible harm can result from prenatal exposure to medications.

   a. **Teratogenicity**—gross organ malformation occurring during the first trimester

   b. **Perinatal syndromes**—neonatal toxicity or withdrawal symptoms within the first few days of life

   c. **Behavioral teratogenicity**—the enduring impact of prenatal exposure on behavior and psychological development

C. FDA pregnancy categories. No psychotropic medication is absolutely safe in pregnancy. All diffuse across the placenta, and most are considered to fall into pregnancy category B or C.

1. **Category A:** Controlled studies in women fail to demonstrate a risk to the fetus. The possibility of fetal harm appears remote.

2. **Category B:** Either animal reproduction studies have not demonstrated fetal risk with no controlled studies in pregnant women, or animal reproduction studies have shown an adverse effect that was not confirmed in controlled studies on women in the first trimester (with no evidence of risk in later trimesters).

3. **Category C:** Either studies in animals have revealed adverse effects on the fetus and there are no controlled studies in women, or studies in women and animals are not available. Drugs in this category should be given only if the potential benefit justifies the risk to the fetus.

4. **Category D:** There is positive evidence of human fetal risk, but the benefits for pregnant women may be acceptable despite this risk.

5. **Category X:** Studies in animals or humans have demonstrated fetal abnormalities, there is evidence of fetal risk based on human experience, or both, and the risk of using the drug in pregnant women clearly outweighs any possible benefit.

D. Risks associated with specific psychotropic medications in pregnancy (see Table 29-1)

III **POSTPARTUM.** Psychiatric disorders that originate during the postpartum period can be divided into three categories:

A. Postpartum blues are estimated to occur in about half of women following delivery and are characterized by symptoms occurring within a few days postpartum and **persisting less than 2**

TABLE 29-1. Risks and Tolerability Associated with Specific Psychotropic Medications in Pregnancy

Agent	Comments
Antipsychotics	The lower potency antipsychotics [e.g., chlorpromazine (Thorazine) and thioridazine (Mellaril)] are generally better tolerated than the higher potency antipsychotics [e.g., haloperidol (Haldol)]. There are minimal data on atypical antipsychotics.
Antidepressants	
Tricyclics	Relatively safe but may be difficult to tolerate because of anticholinergic side effects
SSRIs	Better tolerated than tricyclics and appear to be relatively safe in pregnancy
MAO inhibitors	Cause congenital abnormalities and orthostatic hypotension
Mood Stabilizers	
Lithium	Associated with a 10–20 time increased risk of Ebstein's anomaly (risk in general population is 1 in 20,000) in fetus
Carbamazepine	Associated with up to a 1% rate of spina bifida
Valproic acid	Associated with a 3%–5% risk of neural tube defects in fetus. The combination of carbamazepine (Depakote) and valproate is a stronger teratogen than either alone.
Anxiolytics	
Benzodiazepines	Associated with oral clefts in fetus, especially diazepam (Valium)

SSRIs = selective serotonin reuptake inhibitors; *MAO* = monoamine oxidase.

weeks, including: mood lability, tearfulness, generalized anxiety, and sleep and appetite disturbance. Symptoms are benign and transient and require no specific treatment.

B. Postpartum depression (PPD) is estimated to occur at a rate of about 10%. Women at greatest risk are those with a previous history of a mood disorder or those who experienced depression during the pregnancy.

1. **Clinical manifestations.** Symptoms usually are seen within the first month after delivery but can be seen up to 1 year postpartum. The presentation of a patient with PPD is simi-

lar to that of one with major depressive disorder (see Chapter 15 V B), but often anxiety and obsessional thoughts will be more prominent.

   2. Treatment. For mild to moderate PPD, interpersonal psychotherapy or cognitive-behavioral psychotherapy has been shown to be efficacious. Nonpharmacological methods should be considered, especially if the patient wishes to breastfeed, given the potential for psychiatric medications to enter the breast milk. If pharmacological treatment is necessary, it should be as for a nonpostpartum episode of depression.

C. Postpartum psychosis occurs in about 0.01% to 0.02% of mothers.

   1. Clinical manifestations. The onset is often abrupt, occurring within 48–72 hours postpartum. The patient may present initially with restlessness, irritability, and sleep disturbance, but usually symptoms evolve rapidly into depressed or elevated mood, disorganized behavior, mood lability, delusions, and hallucinations. It is important to rule out psychosis due to a general medical condition (e.g., thyroid disease) and substance-induced psychosis.

   2. Treatment. Postpartum psychosis is a psychiatric emergency requiring inpatient treatment with mood stabilizers, antipsychotics, or ECT. The risk for infanticide with postpartum psychosis is as high as 4%. In the absence of any psychiatric history, postpartum psychosis is often the first episode of a recurrent affective disorder.

References

Altshuler LL, Cohen LS, Szuba MP, et al: Pharmacologic management of psychiatric illness during pregnancy: Dilemmas and guidelines. *Am J Psychiatry* 153(5): 592–606, 1996.

Chaudron LH, Jefferson JW: Mood stabilizers during breastfeeding: A review. *J Clin Psychiatry* 61(2):79–90, 2000.

Cohen LS, Altshuler LL: Pharmacologic management of psychiatric illness during pregnancy and the postpartum period. *Psychiatr Clin North Am* 4:21–60, 1997.

PART X

EATING DISORDERS

30. Anorexia Nervosa

I INTRODUCTION

A. **Definition.** Both anorexia nervosa and bulimia nervosa (see Chapter 31) are characterized by a **disturbance in perception of body shape and weight** and **an intense fear of becoming fat.** Anorexia nervosa is also characterized by a patient's **refusal to maintain a minimally normal body weight.** Symptoms of anorexia nervosa and bulimia nervosa may overlap. The two disorders are often viewed as part of a continuum.

B. **Demographics and incidence**
   1. Eating disorders are found predominantly in women (90%–95% of cases). The prevalence of anorexia nervosa among adolescent and young adult women is estimated at around 1%.
   2. In the past, white, upper-middle-class adolescents and young adult students were the populations most frequently diagnosed with eating disorders. Increasingly, men (especially homosexual men) and women of other racial, socioeconomic, and age groups are being diagnosed.
   3. The overall incidence of eating disorders appears to be increasing.
   4. The incidence of eating disorders is thought to be greater in industrialized countries.

C. **Causes. The etiology of anorexia nervosa is multifactorial.**
   1. **Familial risk factors.** Monozygotic twins of patients with anorexia nervosa have a 50% concordance rate for the disorder, compared with 10% for dizygotic twins and other siblings. There is an increased risk of mood disorders in first-degree relatives of patients with anorexia nervosa.
   2. **Psychological and societal risk factors**
      a. Psychologically, an eating disorder often develops as an attempt by the patient to gain a sense of control in her life, which she otherwise lacks.
      b. Patients with eating disorders may have difficulty in tolerating feelings and interpreting inner physical sensations, such as hunger.

   c. Poor self-esteem and an all-or-nothing style of thinking
      are often seen.
   d. Early histories are often significant for losses or traumas.
   e. Certain characteristics of family functioning may serve as
      a risk factor for eating disorders, such as family function-
      ing in which autonomy is discouraged.
   f. Societal pressure to be thin may also play a role.

 PROFILE Sue is a 15-year-old straight-A student and regional ice skating champion who lives with her domineering mother. Sue
began to diet and lost 5 pounds prior to an important skating competition. She received a great deal of attention and
approval from others for her slim figure.

D. Prognosis
   1. One study showed that after 5–10 years, 50% of patients
      treated for anorexia had a good outcome, 25% were im-
      proved, and 25% either did not improve or had died. Mor-
      tality rates may reach as high as 20% 20 years after first de-
      veloping the disorder, due to complications of anorexia
      nervosa or suicide.
   2. Unfortunately, even among patients who have done well
      with respect to the symptoms of their anorexia nervosa, a
      majority continues to have preoccupations with food and
      body image. Many develop symptoms of bulimia nervosa,
      anxiety, depression, or substance use disorders.

II CLINICAL MANIFESTATIONS

A. Types. Anorexia nervosa can be either of two types:
   1. The **restricting type,** marked by an absence of either binge
      eating or purging. Weight loss is accomplished through diet-
      ing, fasting, or excessive exercise.
   2. The **binge eating/purging type.**
B. Diagnostic criteria for anorexia nervosa can be recalled by the
   mnemonic "DINE."
C. Medical complications of eating disorders can be serious and life-
   threatening. Associated conditions and findings may include:
   —**Electrolyte imbalances** (e.g., hypokalemia secondary to purg-
      ing, hypochloremic metabolic acidosis secondary to vomiting,
      hypomagnesemia, hyperamylasemia), dehydration, edema
   —**Cardiovascular problems** (e.g., arrhythmias secondary to hy-
      pokalemia, hypotension and bradycardia seen with starva-
      tion, cardiomyopathy secondary to ipecac toxicity)
   —**Gastrointestinal complications** (e.g., Mallory-Weiss tears,

Diagnostic Criteria for Anorexia Nervosa ("DINE")

Distorted sense of body shape or weight or undue influence of body shape or weight on self-evaluation, or **De**nial of the seriousness of low body weight
Intense fear of gaining weight
Normal weight **n**ot maintained or gained during growth (patient is less than 85% of normal weight for age and height)
Endocrine abnormalities—missing three consecutive menstrual cycles

esophagitis and parotitis secondary to vomiting; delayed gastric emptying seen with starvation)
—**Dental caries** secondary to vomiting
—**Menstrual irregularities,** especially with bulimia; amenorrhea, especially with anorexia
—**Dermatologic changes** (e.g., callus on dorsum of hand and petechiae from induced vomiting, lanugo hair development)
—**Anemia** (seen with starvation)
—**Nonspecific electroencephalogram (EEG) changes** (seen with starvation)

PROFILE

Sue, the 15-year-old ice skating champion, gradually began to hear from others that she appeared to be "too thin," although she herself felt "fat." Sue began to limit her food intake more aggressively and to avoid foods with certain fat content. She stopped menstruating, and when her weight dropped to 78 pounds, her coach suggested she see a psychiatrist.

III DIFFERENTIAL DIAGNOSIS AND PSYCHIATRIC COMORBIDITIES

A. The **differential diagnosis** of anorexia nervosa includes the following:
   1. Weight loss because of medical conditions, such as acquired immune deficiency syndrome (AIDS), tuberculosis, or cancer
   2. Starvation because of limited external resources
   3. Bulimia nervosa, purging type (see Chapter 31)
   4. Depressive disorders

HOT KEY

Behavioral correlates of starvation may appear to represent a depressive disorder. Careful assessment is required to rule out a comorbid or primary depressive disorder.

a. Symptoms of decreased food intake, withdrawal, depressed or irritable mood, obsessive ruminations, poor concentration, insomnia, and lack of interest in sex **suggest depression but may in fact be directly related to the state of starvation.** Starvation-related symptoms will remit with weight gain.

b. Features that are useful in distinguishing a depressive disorder from anorexia are outlined in Table 30-1.

TABLE 30-1. Distinguishing Features of Anorexia Nervosa and Depression

Criteria or feature	Anorexia	Depression
Fear of weight gain and distorted sense of one's body shape	Present	Absent
Appetite	Patients have normal or increased appetites until late stages	Decreased
Self-esteem	Highly focused on weight and body image	Impaired in many areas
Obsessive rumination	Focused on food	Focused on guilty themes

5. Psychosis (paranoid or bizarre delusions about food, the body, or food servers, or related to marked negative symptoms, e.g., a psychotic patient who believes that others are conspiring to poison him may persistently refuse food)
6. Somatization disorder (see Chapter 27 II C 5)
7. Conversion disorder with psychogenic vomiting (see Chapter 27 II C 1)
8. Social phobia (see Chapter 19 II A)
9. Body dysmorphic disorder (see Chapter 27 II C 2)
B. Psychiatric comorbidities
   1. There is an increased incidence of **depressive and anxiety disorders** in patients with eating disorders. Up to 50%–75% of patients with anorexia nervosa may also have a depressive disorder.

2. **Obsessive–compulsive disorder** (OCD). Obsessions and compulsions unrelated to food may suggest comorbid OCD. The lifetime prevalence of OCD in patients with anorexia may be up to 25%.

3. Patients with binge eating/purging type are more likely to have other **impulsive tendencies** (e.g., shoplifting, sexual promiscuity, and affective lability) and are more likely to have **borderline personality disorder.**

IV APPROACH TO THE PATIENT

A. **Medical complications** of eating disorders can be serious and life-threatening.

1. A **full medical history** should be taken, including information about the patient's menstrual history (if the patient is female).

2. A **complete physical examination** is also essential, as complications of anorexia may manifest themselves in almost any organ system (see II C). It is important to include vital signs with orthostatic blood pressures, height, weight, and staging of sexual development.

3. **Laboratory studies** should include, at a minimum, a complete blood cell (CBC) count, electrolytes, blood urea nitrogen (BUN), creatinine, and a urinalysis. If indicated, thyroid function tests (TFTs), liver function tests (LFTs), amylase, carotene, calcium, magnesium, phosphorus, zinc, and an electrocardiogram (EKG) should be performed.

4. **Consultation** may be required with specialists in nutrition, dentistry, pediatrics, general internal medicine, endocrinology, cardiology, or gastroenterology.

B. A **full psychiatric history** should also be taken to assess for potential comorbid psychiatric conditions.

1. The evaluation should include a longitudinal assessment of the patient's eating and compensatory behaviors and body image.

2. Family attitudes and behaviors surrounding food and body image should be explored.

V TREATMENT

A. **Outpatient treatment.** Patients with anorexia nervosa can often be treated as outpatients.

1. Treatment is initially focused on physiologically stabilizing the patient. This often involves monitoring food intake, weight, and relevant laboratory indices and determining target weights and a behavioral treatment plan regarding eating and weight gain.

2. Nutritional rehabilitation needs to be carefully planned, as overly rapid re-feeding can lead to cardiac failure.

B. Psychotherapy

1. Psychotherapy may initially focus on psychoeducation and supportive and behavioral interventions. **The patient may not understand that her eating behaviors are problematic.**
2. After the patient is stabilized physiologically, treatment may focus on **psychological, interpersonal, family,** or other issues.
3. Various psychotherapeutic approaches may be invoked, including cognitive or psychoanalytic treatments.
4. In order to build a rapport with the patient, it is important that the physician be **firm** and **nonjudgmental.**

HOT ▶ **KEY** The patient must regard the physician as someone who is interested in ameliorating the suffering caused by her underlying psychological problems and not just interested in convincing her to eat.

---

5. Family therapy can be very helpful, especially if the patient is an adolescent.

PROFILE Sue was ultimately hospitalized on an inpatient psychiatric unit where, after several months of behavioral treatment and individual and family psychotherapy, she gained 12 pounds and was discharged to home.

In her therapy, Sue is working on identifying her own feelings and desires, accepting herself as she is, and learning to take more active control of the decisions that affect her life.

C. Pharmacotherapy plays a **limited role** in treating anorexia nervosa.

1. Antidepressants should be considered if depressive symptoms do not improve with normalization of weight. Tricyclic antidepressants may place the patient at increased risk for arrhythmias and hypotension.
2. Low-dose antipsychotic medications are sometimes used for psychotic-like thinking in anorexia nervosa.
3. Short-acting benzodiazepines may be useful 1 hour prior to meals if a patient experiences significant anxiety at mealtimes.
4. Medications that speed the rate of gastric emptying may be useful in some cases to prevent the patient from purging or to prevent the feeling of fullness.

D. Hospitalization. Patients may need inpatient admission if out-patient treatment is not effective, weight drops more than 30% below normal, significant medical complications occur, or suicidality is a concern.

References

American Psychiatric Association Work Group on Eating Disorders: Practice guideline for the treatment of patients with eating disorders (revision). *Am J Psychiatry* 157(suppl 1):1–39, 2000.

Brown JM, Mehler PS, Harris RH: Medical complications occurring in adolescents with anorexia nervosa. *West J Med* 172(3):189–193, 2000.

Pike KM: Long-term course of anorexia nervosa: Response, relapse, remission, and recovery. *Clin Psychol Rev* 18(4):447–475, 1998.

Walsh BT, Devlin MJ: Eating disorders: Progress and problems. *Science* 280(5368) May 29:1387–1390, 1998.

31. Bulimia Nervosa

I INTRODUCTION

A. Definition. As with anorexia nervosa, bulimia nervosa is marked by a **disturbance in perception of body shape and weight** and **an intense fear of becoming fat.** Binge eating occurs, usually involving foods with high carbohydrate and fat content. **Compensatory behaviors following binge-eating episodes** may include self-induced vomiting; using laxatives, diuretics, or enemas; fasting; or excessive exercising.

B. Demographics
   1. The demographics for bulimia nervosa are much like those for anorexia nervosa:
      a. It predominantly affects women (90%–95%).
      b. Traditionally, white upper-middle-class adolescents and young adult students who live in industrialized countries have been the majority of patients.
      c. The overall incidence of this disorder is increasing, and men as well as women from other racial, socioeconomic, and age groups are increasingly affected.
   2. The prevalence of adolescent and young adult women who fulfill criteria for bulimia nervosa is about 2%. This rate is higher than that of anorexia nervosa.

HOT KEY

Whereas patients with anorexia nervosa are underweight, patients with bulimia nervosa may be of normal weight, overweight, or slightly underweight.

C. Causes. The etiology is multifactorial.
   1. **Familial risk factors.** Monozygotic twins of patients with bulimia nervosa have a higher incidence of the disorder than dizygotic twins, which is higher than the general population. In first-degree relatives of patients with bulimia nervosa, there appears to be an increased risk of bulimia nervosa, mood disorders, substance abuse and dependence, and possibly obesity.
   2. **Neurotransmitter abnormalities.** Some research suggests that a deficiency in central serotonin may play a role.
   3. **Psychological and societal risk factors.** As with anorexia ner-

vosa, the behaviors of bulimia nervosa may be viewed as an attempt by the patient to gain a sense of control in her life or may be related to **difficulty tolerating affect** and **interpreting inner sensations.** Also as with anorexia nervosa, **poor self-esteem** and an **all-or-nothing style of thinking** are often seen and early histories are often significant for losses or traumas; certain characteristics of family functioning may serve as a risk factor for eating disorders, and societal pressures for thinness may play a role.

D. Prognosis
1. Bulimia nervosa tends to follow **highly variable waxing and waning courses** with symptoms reemerging during periods of stress in the patient's life. Long-term remissions are possible.
2. Mortality risk is unknown. Roughly 70% of those treated as outpatients have shown a significant improvement in symptoms and maintained their gains over several years, although with some symptoms persisting. Patients requiring hospitalization tend to have a worse prognosis.

II CLINICAL MANIFESTATIONS

A. Types. Bulimia nervosa is either of the **purging type** (use of vomiting, laxatives, diuretics, or enemas) or **nonpurging type** (use of fasting or excessive exercise).

B. Diagnostic criteria for bulimia nervosa can be recalled by the mnemonic "BINGE."

Diagnostic Criteria for Bulimia Nervosa ("BINGE")

Binge eating: ingesting a large amount of food over a discrete period of time while lacking a sense of control
Inappropriate influence of body shape and weight on self-evaluation
No less than twice per week for 3 months (both binge eating and purging)
Gain (of weight) prevented by compensatory behaviors
Exclusion criteria—does not occur exclusively during anorexia nervosa episodes

MNEMONIC

C. Medical complications. The complications of bulimia nervosa can involve many body systems and can be serious and life-threatening (see Chapter 30 II C).

III DIFFERENTIAL DIAGNOSIS AND PSYCHIATRIC COMORBIDITIES

A. The **differential diagnoses** of bulimia nervosa include the following:
1. Anorexia nervosa, binge eating/purging type
2. Major depressive disorder with atypical features
3. Complex partial seizures
4. Medical or central nervous system (CNS) pathology leading to binge eating and vomiting
5. Klüver-Bucy syndrome
6. Kleine-Levin syndrome

B. Comorbid psychiatric conditions for patients with bulimia nervosa are significant and should be carefully assessed.
1. Patients with bulimia nervosa are at highly increased risk for **depressive** or **anxiety disorders.** These disorders may begin before, concurrent with, or after the onset of the bulimia.
2. Up to 50% of patients with bulimia nervosa may also have a **personality disorder.** Borderline type is a particularly frequent comorbid personality disorder.
3. Up to 50% of individuals with bulimia nervosa also suffer from **alcohol or stimulant abuse or dependence.**
4. Twenty to fifty percent of patients with bulimia nervosa may have a **history of sexual abuse.**
5. **Dissociative symptoms** and **impulsive behaviors** (e.g., shoplifting, sexual promiscuity) also occur more frequently in patients with bulimia.

IV APPROACH TO THE PATIENT.
The medical and psychiatric approach to the patient with bulimia nervosa is similar to that for a patient with anorexia nervosa (see Chapter 30 IV).

V TREATMENT

A. Outpatient treatment. Most patients with bulimia can be treated as outpatients. As with anorexia, treatment is often initially focused on **physiologically stabilizing the patient and determining behavioral goals and contingencies.**

B. Psychotherapy
1. The physician should be **firm** and **nonjudgmental,** and the psychotherapy may initially focus on psychoeducation and supportive and behavioral interventions.
2. After the patient is stabilized physiologically, treatment may focus on psychological, interpersonal, family, or other issues, with other psychotherapeutic approaches invoked.
3. Patients with bulimia nervosa tend to be more distressed by

their symptoms than patients with anorexia nervosa, yet it is still **important to work on the underlying psychological problems rather than just the eating behaviors.**
   a. **Cognitive-behavioral therapy** may be more useful than other approaches in treating bulimia nervosa.
   b. Family therapy can play an important role, especially if the patient is an adolescent.
   c. Group therapy can often be particularly useful.
C. Pharmacological treatment, most notably with antidepressants, can be useful in decreasing the frequency of binge eating and purging. Desipramine, imipramine, and trazodone may be administered in standard doses, and fluoxetine in doses up to 60 mg. Monoamine oxidase inhibitors (MAOIs) may be useful if the patient can adhere to the dietary restrictions.
D. Hospitalization. Inpatient treatment or day hospital treatment may be indicated for symptoms unresponsive to outpatient management, suicidal crises, life-threatening medical complications, or severe concurrent substance abuse.

References

American Psychiatric Association Work Group on Eating Disorders: Practice guideline for the treatment of patients with eating disorders (revision). *Am J Psychiatry* 157(suppl 1):1–39, 2000.

Kaye WH, Klump KL, Frank GK, et al: Anorexia and bulimia nervosa. *Ann Rev Med* 51:299–313, 2000.

Keel PK, Mitchell JE: Outcome in bulimia nervosa. *Am J Psychiatry* 154(3):313–321, 1997.

Mcgilley BM, Pryor TL: Assessment and treatment of bulimia nervosa. *Am Fam Physician* 57(11):2743–2750, 1998.

PART XI

SLEEP AND ITS DISORDERS

•••

32. Normal Sleep
....

I **INTRODUCTION.** Sleep is an active physiologic process with discrete states during which specific bodily functions, and probably mental functions, occur. To better understand sleep abnormalities, it is important to learn the basics of normal sleep. Sleep can be evaluated using a **polysomnogram** with the simultaneous recording of:

A. Brain activity [electroencephalogram (EEG) channels]
B. Eye movements (electro-oculogram)
C. Muscle tone and movement [chin, arm, and leg electromyogram (EMG)]
D. Cardiac function (electrocardiogram)
E. Respiratory effort and airflow

II **STATES OF SLEEP.** As a person falls asleep, the brain cycles through two states of sleep: **rapid eye movement (REM) and non-rapid eye movement (NREM) sleep.**

A. NREM sleep occurs first in a normal adult, with the brain going into **successively deeper levels or stages** (Table 32-1).
   1. During NREM sleep, muscle tone and deep tendon reflexes are present and bodily repositioning takes place approximately every 15 minutes.
   2. Heart rate and blood pressure fall to their lowest levels but remain regular.
   3. The pulsatile release of growth hormone occurs within the first hour of NREM sleep.
   4. When awakened from NREM sleep, people may recall simple mentation. However, arousing from the deepest stages of NREM sleep is typically accompanied by several minutes of disorientation.
B. REM sleep begins 90–120 minutes after the onset of NREM sleep and has a very different physiology. REM sleep is when most dreams occur, so it is also called "dreaming sleep."
   1. An EEG of REM (or dreaming sleep) is similar to that of a

TABLE 32-1. Stages of Non-Rapid Eye Movement (NREM) Sleep	
NREM Stage	**Characteristics**
1	Lightest sleep EEG loses the alpha activity (i.e., 8–12 Hz) characteristic of an awake brain with eyes closed and begins to show theta activity (i.e., 3–7 Hz) EMG tone is reduced and slow, rolling eye movements are present; vertex sharp waves are occasionally seen
2	EEG shows progressive slowing with prominent theta activity (3–7 Hz); brief, spindle-shaped bursts of fast activity (i.e., sleep spindles; 12–14 Hz); and slow, high-voltage triphasic waves (i.e., K complexes)
3	EEG shows appearance of slow waves (i.e., delta waves; 0.5–2.0 Hz) mixed with theta activity; spindles and K complexes may or may not be present
4	Deepest sleep EEG shows mostly delta waves

EEG = electroencephalogram; *EMG* = electromyogram.

waking brain, with low-voltage fast activity. However, an EEG of dreaming sleep also has characteristic sawtooth waves.

2. During REM sleep, the eyes show bursts of conjugate horizontal movement (i.e., rapid eye movements). The function of these eye movements is unclear, but they do not reliably reflect dream activity.

3. During REM sleep, only the diaphragm and extraocular muscles can move.

4. Heart rate and blood pressure are variable and erratic during REM sleep, a factor contributing to the increased incidence of myocardial infarction in the early waking hours.

5. During REM sleep, thermoregulation is not engaged (i.e., physiology becomes poikilothermic).

6. When awakened from REM sleep, dreams are usually recalled as complex and richly visual.

HOT KEY ▶ Deep tendon reflexes and muscle tone are absent during REM sleep because the brain evokes a flaccid paralysis of the skeletal muscles, probably to prevent dreams from being acted out.

C. NREM and REM stages continue to occur in an **alternating cyclic pattern** approximately every 90 minutes.
   1. **As sleep continues, episodes of NREM sleep continue to get shorter and lighter and episodes of REM sleep get longer.**
   2. Delta sleep or slow-wave sleep (i.e., NREM stages 3 and 4; see Table 32-1) usually occurs in the first third of the night.
   3. The first episode of REM sleep is only several minutes long, but by morning REM episodes may last for 1 hour or longer, and dreaming activity is typically more vivid (Figure 32-1).

III CIRCADIAN RHYTHM. When people are placed in an isolated environment that is free of any indicators of time, sleep and wakefulness begin to occur in regular intervals that span close to a 24-hour period. This cyclic variation in rest and activity is called the **endogenous circadian rhythm,** and it is seen in all animals and plants.

A. Circadian rhythm appears to guide sleep-wake cycles, core body temperature, serum cortisol levels, and other physiologic parameters.
B. An individual's circadian rhythm is preprogrammed (genetically) through the pacemaker, the **suprachiasmatic nucleus.** This rhythm, though, can be influenced by some external factors.
   1. Connections from the retina, and possibly other body areas, allow exposure to light to stimulate the suprachiasmatic nucleus to start "daytime" or wakefulness in humans.
   2. **Melatonin** is a hormone that is synthesized by the pineal gland and released in darkness (i.e., the "dark hormone"). It appears to help the suprachiasmatic nucleus maintain a coherent circadian rhythm by cueing nighttime.
C. To adapt to the 24-hour world that we live in, every day our brains are entrained by the day-night cycle and social cues (called zeitgebers) that govern our daily routines (e.g., eating breakfast at a regular time).

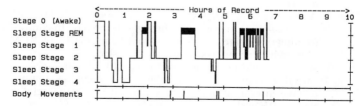

FIGURE 32-1. Hypnogram showing sleep pattern recorded in a healthy young adult. (From Kaplan HI, Sadock BJ (eds): *Comprehensive Textbook of Psychiatry,* 6th ed. Baltimore, Williams & Wilkins, 1995.)

HOT KEY Many people take melatonin to help them get to sleep because of its importance in sleep regulation. However, melatonin has not been rigorously evaluated for insomnia, and its long-term safety is unknown. Pregnant women and children should not use melatonin.

D. Subjective sleepiness levels are always greatest at night because of our circadian clocks. However, there is also a significant period of sleepiness in the afternoon from 2–4 P.M. (i.e., the "siesta" period).

HOT KEY Driving accidents caused by motorists who fall asleep and accidents that occur while performing work that requires sustained vigilance occur most frequently at night and during the "siesta" period. Unfortunately, many lectures in universities occur during the midafternoon period of heightened sleepiness.

IV **SLEEP FUNCTIONS.** Although there is speculation, the function of sleep is still unclear. Probable functions include:

A. Growth and maintenance of normal physiologic functions
B. Consolidation of memories (attributed to REM sleep)
C. Energy conservation

V **SLEEP REQUIREMENTS**

A. The amount of sleep required differs from person to person and changes across the life span.

   1. A 28-week-old fetus shows sleep-wake patterns that are regular, with most of the sleep in REM. Twenty hours or more are spent in sleep, punctuated by waking activity (movement).

   2. A neonate sleeps an average of 16–20 hours each day, with sleep occurring in segments throughout the day. In contrast to adults, neonates go directly from being awake to REM sleep, which accounts for 50% of their sleep.

   3. A young child (2–5 years old) needs 10–12 hours of sleep each day. Young children usually sleep at night but continue to take afternoon naps. Thirty percent of a young child's sleep is REM sleep.

   4. A teenager (13–18 years old) needs an average of 9 hours of sleep at night. During the teen years, the circadian rhythm shifts temporarily to favor falling asleep at later hours, often making it difficult for teens to awaken easily in time for school. Also, the increased release of gonadotropins that guide puberty occurs largely during sleep.

5. An adult (19 years old and over) typically needs 7–8 hours of sleep each day; however, some individuals need as little as 4–5 hours or as much as 10–12 hours. REM sleep accounts for 20%–25% of an adult's sleep.

6. Elderly adults (over 60 years old) need approximately 6–8 hours of sleep each day. However, their sleep is often more fragmented and lighter due to the development of medical problems, medication side effects, or sleep disorders.

B. Sleep is strongly influenced by many other factors, including:

1. Amount of prior sleep deprivation (sleep will be longer with more slow waves in recovery from more than a few hours of sleep deprivation)

2. Illness and physical or emotional stress

3. Exercise (increases slow-wave sleep)

4. Medications currently taken and medication withdrawal

5. Alcohol, nicotine, and caffeine (current use or withdrawal state)

6. Exposure to light (i.e., seasonal changes)

7. Motivation, social interaction, and activity levels

References

Kahn A, Dan B, Groswasser J, et al: Normal sleep architecture in infants and children. *J Clin Neurophysiol* 13(3):184–197, 1996.

Prinz PN: Sleep and sleep disorders in older adults. *J Clin Neurophysiol* 12(2):139–146, 1995.

Sack RL, Hughes RJ, Edgar DM, et al: Sleep-promoting effects of melatonin: At what dose, in whom, under what conditions, and by what mechanisms? *Sleep* 20(10):908–915, 1997.

33. Sleep Disorders

I **INTRODUCTION.** Sleep disorders can take many forms. The **most common sleep disorder is insomnia,** which is discussed in detail in **Chapter 34. This chapter focuses on other common causes of sleep disturbance that are frequently overlooked in the clinical setting.**

II **CLINICAL MANIFESTATIONS OF SLEEP DISORDERS.**
Some sleep disorders, such as sleepwalking, are not difficult to diagnose when someone has witnessed the episode. However, some of the most common sleep disorders do not present with clearly identifiable symptoms.

A. Symptoms of **excessive daytime sleepiness** should alert the physician to the possibility of a sleep disorder.
   1. When sleep is disrupted significantly, the physiologic pressure to sleep builds and it becomes more and more difficult to remain fully alert. This may result in an intense desire to sleep.
   2. However, many people are not consciously aware of the degree of sleepiness they are struggling with because of an occult sleep disorder. This is especially true if the sleep disorder developed gradually, with efforts to compensate for it made slowly over time.
B. Excessive sleepiness can result in the following **mood or physical problems:**
   1. Memory and concentration problems
   2. Depressed or irritable mood
   3. Decreased energy
   4. Decreased libido
   5. Yawning
   6. Red, irritated eyes
C. Sleepiness is more likely to manifest as falling asleep during sedentary activities such as reading, watching television, or riding as a passenger in a vehicle. If frequent, this degree of sleepiness is **not normal.**

HOT **KEY**
Dozing while driving or during a conversation are signs of serious impairment due to sleepiness.

III **CLASSIFICATION OF SLEEP DISORDERS.** There are approximately 80 recognized sleep disorders, each with a different cause. It is helpful to classify sleep disorders as **dyssomnias** (i.e., abnormalities in the amount, quality, or timing of sleep), **parasomnias** (i.e., abnormal behaviors or physiologic events that occur during sleep-wake transitions), and sleep disorders due to an **underlying medical or psychiatric condition.**

HOT

The most common cause of pathologic levels of daytime sleepiness in the general population is sleep deprivation.

KEY

A. **Dyssomnias**
  1. **Obstructive sleep apnea syndrome (OSAS)**
     a. OSAS occurs when the **upper airway collapses or becomes obstructed during sleep,** preventing airflow (i.e., apnea). The loss of airflow, development of hypoxia, or both then trigger an awakening from sleep, which restores breathing. Once breathing is reestablished, sleep resumes and the airway can again become obstructed. In severe cases, this cycle of apnea-arousal can occur 700 times or more each night.
     b. There are many potential causes of airway collapse during sleep. The most common causes include:
        (1) Overcrowded oropharynx (e.g., large uvula or tonsils)
        (2) Obesity (fat pads around the airway result in a narrowing of the airway)
        (3) Retrognathia (which leads to a smaller upper airway)
        (4) Hypothyroidism and hyperandrogenism (both cause enlargement of airway muscles)
     c. The consequences of OSAS are **severely fragmented sleep** and significant time during sleep spent with **inadequate oxygenation.** Both contribute to the substantial morbidity and mortality of this syndrome.
     d. In addition to excessive daytime sleepiness, the long-term sequelae of untreated OSAS include **risk of hypertension, arrhythmia, and cor pulmonale.**
  2. **Central sleep apnea syndrome (CSAS)**
     a. CSAS is defined as repetitive apnea caused by the intermittent cessation of the drive to breathe. CSAS is much less common than OSAS.
     b. The consequences of CSAS are similar to those of OSAS.
  3. **Periodic limb movement disorder**
     a. Periodic limb movement disorder is characterized by

repetitive (i.e., every 20–40 seconds) leg or arm twitches that cause frequent arousals from sleep. Although the patient may not be aware of the kicking or jerking movements, bed partners may be aware of the movements.

b. The underlying cause is unknown. It is often present in older individuals with underlying medical problems such as peripheral neuropathy, circulatory disorders, arthritis, and iron deficiency anemia.

4. Restless legs syndrome

   a. Restless legs syndrome is an **unbearable restless feeling** in the legs that is relieved by movement. It begins during the early evening hours, making sedentary activities (e.g., watching television) difficult.

   b. Sleep onset is delayed because the patient cannot remain still in bed.

   c. Most people who complain of restless legs syndrome also have periodic limb movement disorder on polysomnogram testing.

> **HOT** ▶ **KEY**   Tricyclic antidepressants (TCAs), selective serotonin reuptake inhibitors (SSRIs), and monoamine oxidase inhibitors (MAOIs) can cause periodic limb movement disorder and restless legs syndrome.

5. Narcolepsy

   a. Narcolepsy is a neurologic disorder of sleep-wake regulation of unknown etiology.

   b. **Excessive daytime sleepiness** is the primary symptom and may be severely disabling. Other associated symptoms include:

   (1) Cataplexy [brief (1–2 minute) episodes of muscle weakness are triggered by strong emotions (e.g., laughter, surprise, sexual excitement)]. A patient is awake and aware during cataplexy, even if her eyes are closed.

   (2) Frequent hypnagogic hallucinations

   (3) Frequent episodes of sleep paralysis

   (4) Disrupted nocturnal sleep

   c. Genetic factors predispose individuals to narcolepsy.

6. Circadian rhythm disorders

   a. Circadian rhythm disorders are characterized by a tendency to fall asleep at the "wrong" time.

   (1) Delayed sleep phase disorder presents with difficulty falling asleep before the early morning hours and difficulty awakening before midday (i.e., "night owl").

    (2) Advanced sleep phase disorder presents with a tendency to fall asleep early in the evening and awaken early in the morning (i.e., "a lark").

  b. People with circadian rhythm disorders do not usually have mood disorders or other sleep complaints but may describe themselves as "insomniacs" because of their odd sleep hours.

B. Parasomnias

1. Nightmares

  a. Nightmares are frightening dreams that are recalled in vivid detail. Nightmares **occur during rapid eye movement (REM) sleep.**

  b. Nightmares often accompany depressive or posttraumatic episodes and may be evoked by alcohol withdrawal or treatment with β-blockers.

2. Night-terrors

  a. Night-terrors are characterized by partial arousal from non-rapid eye movement (NREM) sleep with **exaggerated autonomic arousal,** giving the appearance of terror (e.g., screaming, palpitations, rapid breathing, diaphoresis). At the time of partial arousal, patients do not recall any clear dream detail. In the morning, patients often do not recall the episode.

  b. Night-terrors occur most often during the transition from stage 3 to stage 2 sleep (see Table 32-1) [i.e., during the first few hours of sleep].

  c. Although the occurrence of night-terrors is common and considered "normal" in children, it can be correlated with stress or psychopathology in adults.

3. Somnambulism (i.e., sleepwalking)

  a. Somnambulism is characterized by walking or other behaviors while still apparently asleep.

  b. Like night-terrors, somnambulism occurs during the first few hours of sleep (i.e., NREM sleep).

  c. Somnambulism is common in children and may be precipitated by sedating medications [e.g., **zolpidem** (Ambien)] or alcohol in adults.

4. REM sleep behavior disorder

  a. REM sleep behavior disorder is characterized by complex, often violent activities that occur during REM sleep in apparent attempts to enact a dream.

  b. This disorder arises mostly in older men who have damage to the central nervous system centers that initiate the flaccid paralysis that accompanies REM sleep.

C. Sleep disorders due to an underlying medical condition. Some medical problems can cause fatigue, and some nighttime

symptoms of medical problems cause disrupted sleep. These include:

1. Nocturnal asthma
2. Congestive heart failure
3. Uncontrolled pain or hypertension
4. Multiple sclerosis
5. Central nervous system tumors or infections
6. Myotonic dystrophy
7. Other chronic medical conditions (e.g., tuberculosis, thyroid disease, chronic obstructive pulmonary disease)

IV APPROACH TO THE PATIENT

A. To determine the presence of a sleep disorder, it is important to take a thorough **sleep history.** Table 33-1 outlines the basic

TABLE 33-1. Targeted Questions to Include in a Sleep History

Underlying Sleep Pathology	Targeted Questions
Sleep apnea syndrome (obstructive or central)	Do you snore? Has anyone witnessed you gasp or stop breathing during sleep?
Periodic limb movement disorder	Has anyone witnessed kicking or twitching of your limbs during sleep?
Restless legs syndrome	Do you feel restless in the evening before going to sleep? Is the restless feeling relieved by pacing or other movement?
Nightmares	Do you have vivid dreams or nightmares? If so, are they repetitive?
Narcolepsy	As you fall asleep or wake up, do you frequently experience dreamlike hallucinations? Do you ever find yourself unable to move, as if paralyzed, when transitioning from a sleeping state to a waking state?
Enuresis/OSAS	Do you ever urinate during sleep?
Sleepwalking, REM sleep behavior disorder	Do you ever find evidence or have you been told that you have been out of bed during the night without recall?

OSAS = obstructive sleep apnea syndrome; REM = rapid eye movement.

questions addressed in a sleep history. In addition, the targeted questions in Table 33–1 will help to identify the underlying sleep pathology.

B. Although sleep disorders may be initially identified by history, some disorders require evaluation by **polysomnogram.**

C. Daytime polysomnogram testing to objectively evaluate levels of sleepiness during the day may also be necessary.

V TREATMENT

A. **OSAS** is treated using a variety of strategies.
1. Nasal **continuous positive airway pressure (CPAP)** is the most commonly used treatment and is universally effective. A CPAP device uses pressurized air to splint open the airway during sleep.
2. Surgery of the soft palate, uvula, tonsils, and adenoids may also be effective if anatomic defects create obstruction to airflow.
3. When appropriate, weight loss is used to treat OSAS.

B. **CSAS** also may benefit from CPAP or nocturnal ventilation.

C. **Periodic limb movement disorder and restless legs syndrome** often occur together; therefore, the approach to treatment is similar.
1. Medications that suppress limb movements are often effective. Commonly used medications include Sinemet 25/100 (carbidopa and levodopa) and low-dose clonazepam (0.5–1.0 mg) taken at bedtime.
2. Restlessness is effectively treated with gabapentin (100–1500 mg) taken in the evening and at bedtime. Start with 100–300 mg in the evening and increase to 300–900 mg in the evening with repeat doses at bedtime.

D. **Narcolepsy** can be treated with wake-promoting medications and antidepressants.
1. The excessive daytime sleepiness associated with narcolepsy is treated with **wake-promoting medications** (e.g., modafinil, methylphenidate, amphetamines) to restore alertness to functional levels.
2. Cataplexy is suppressed with antidepressants, which reduce REM sleep. TCAs, SSRIs, and MAOIs are all effective.

E. **Nightmares** require treatment of the underlying symptoms of depression, posttraumatic stress disorder, or anxiety.

F. **Night-terrors and sleepwalking** require attention to safety in addition to treatment of the disorder.
1. To make the patient's environment safer, suggest that she lock all doors and windows and install alarms on doors to the outside.
2. When patient safety is a serious concern, the immediate use

of medication is appropriate. A low-dose TCA (e.g., desipramine, 10–50 mg) or benzodiazepine (e.g., diazepam, 2–10 mg) is effective.

3. Sometimes a short course of insight-oriented psychotherapy that allows the patient to express feelings directly is all that is necessary to resolve the sleep behavior.

G. REM sleep behavior disorder also requires attention to safety in addition to pharmacotherapy.

1. It is important to make the patient's environment safer, as you would for sleepwalking, and to protect the patient's bed partner (e.g., sleeping separately).

2. To resolve the behavior, start with low-dose clonazepam (0.5 mg) or a TCA (e.g., desipramine, 10 mg) and increase gradually until the behavior is under control.

VI FOLLOW-UP AND REFERRAL

A. A patient suspected of having a primary sleep disorder that fails initial therapy should be sent to a **sleep disorder center** for further evaluation and treatment.

B. A patient suspected of having significant daytime sleepiness should be cautioned about the risks of driving while drowsy and the additive impact of alcohol and sedatives (including medication) on sleepiness levels.

References

Chokrovery S: Diagnosis and treatment of sleep disorders caused by co-morbid disease. *Neurology* 54(5 suppl 1):S8–15, 2000.

Mahowald MW: What is causing excessive daytime sleepiness? Evaluation to distinguish sleep deprivation from sleep disorders. *Postgrad Med* 107(3):108–110, 115–118, 123, 2000.

Schenck CH, Mahowald MW: Parasomnias: Managing bizarre sleep-related behavior disorders. *Postgrad Med* 107(3):145–156, 2000.

34. Insomnia

I **INTRODUCTION.** Insomnia is **the most common sleep complaint.** It may simply be a manifestation of temporary anxiety (e.g., midterm exam in the morning) or an unpleasant sleep environment (e.g., fraternity house). However, insomnia may also reflect an underlying medical or psychiatric illness, or it may be a side effect of medication used to treat an underlying illness. There are also several sleep disorders that may be experienced as disrupted sleep and require specific interventions other than administration of a sedative-hypnotic (see Chapter 33). Insomnia may be experienced as one or more of the following patterns of sleep disruption:

A. Difficulty falling asleep (initial insomnia)
B. Difficulty maintaining sleep (middle insomnia)
C. Early morning wakening (terminal insomnia)

II **CLINICAL MANIFESTATIONS OF INSOMNIA.** Insomnia causes a feeling of unrefreshing or light sleep. In some cases, people claim to be awake all night, although this is usually not true. As a result of insomnia, people may experience:

A. Fatigue rather than sleepiness during waking hours
B. An inability to nap
C. Problems with mood, concentration, and memory

III **CAUSES OF INSOMNIA.** The onset, duration, and nature of a patient's sleep complaint often indicate the underlying

Common Causes of Insomnia ("INSOMNIAC")

Illness due to a medical condition
Neurologic or psychiatric disease
Sleep disorder
Overconcern about falling asleep
Medications
Noisy or unpleasant sleep environment
Idiopathic causes
Anxiety
Circadian rhythm disruption

cause. Following are general causes to consider when evaluating a patient with insomnia.

A. Insomnia may be a symptom of a **medical illness,** especially if pain or discomfort are present (Table 34-1).

B. **Neurologic and psychiatric diseases** often lead to sleeplessness (Table 34-2).

HOT KEY

Depression is a common cause of insomnia.

C. Patients who present with insomnia may actually be suffering from symptoms of a **primary sleep disorder** that disrupts sleep (see Chapter 33). The presence of an underlying sleep disorder is often accompanied by complaints of excessive daytime sleepiness rather than fatigue.

D. Patients who are **overly concerned about falling asleep** may develop **psychophysiologic insomnia.** When insomnia begins, people frequently become preoccupied with their inability to sleep. Although the initial stressor or cause of insomnia eventually resolves, people remain preoccupied with the inability to sleep.

E. Many **medications** disrupt sleep (Table 34-3).

TABLE 34-1. Medical Disorders That Cause Insomnia

Hyperthyroidism
Uncontrolled hypertension
Uremia
Poorly controlled diabetes (hypoglycemia or hyperglycemia)
Reflux esophagitis
Uncontrolled pain
Nocturia
Addison's disease
Asthma
Fibromyalgia
HIV and AIDS
Withdrawal from alcohol or medications (e.g., antidepressants)
Chronic headache (often during or shortly after REM sleep)
Peptic ulcer disease (gastric secretions increase at night)
Chronic obstructive pulmonary disease (oxygen desaturation is lowest during REM sleep)

AIDS = acquired immune deficiency syndrome; *HIV* = human immunodeficiency virus; *REM* = rapid eye movement.

TABLE 34-2. Psychiatric and Neurologic Disorders That Cause Insomnia

Psychiatric Causes	Neurologic Causes
Mania	CNS infections
Depression	CNS neoplasms
Prodromal schizophrenia	Migraine headache
Acute psychosis	Neuropathic pain
Posttraumatic stress disorder	Neurodegenerative disorders
Dementia	
Anxiety disorders (e.g., obsessive–compulsive disorder, panic disorder, generalized anxiety disorder)	
Eating disorders (including nighttime eating binges)	
Substance abuse (e.g., nicotine*)	
Withdrawal from substances (e.g., alcohol, cocaine, opiates)	

CNS = central nervous system.
*Heavy smokers (i.e., two or more packs per day) often wake up in nicotine withdrawal and need to smoke to be able to return to sleep.

F. Transient sleeplessness often occurs in a **noisy, unfamiliar,** or **unpleasant sleep environment.**

G. In some patients, despite a thorough evaluation, the cause of insomnia remains unclear (i.e., **idiopathic insomnia**). Typically, this disorder begins in childhood.

TABLE 34-3. Common Medications That Cause Insomnia

Nicotine
Caffeine
Alcohol
β-Blockers
Theophylline
Corticosteroids
Opiate analgesics
Bupropion
Selective serotonin reuptake inhibitors
Monoamine oxidase inhibitors
Short-acting hypnotics
Risperidone

H. Insomnia may be a result of **anxiety** related to a stressful event.

I. If sleep schedules are chronically disrupted (e.g., shift work, jet lag), **circadian rhythm** may be impaired, leading to disrupted sleep. It is also common to have difficulty returning to a normal night of sleep after a sleepless night due to work or play.

HOT KEY Many normal life changes in women are accompanied by disrupted sleep. For example, the hormonal fluctuations associated with menstruation, pregnancy, and menopause evoke middle insomnia in some women.

IV **APPROACH TO THE PATIENT.** When approaching a patient with insomnia, keep in mind that **insomnia is a symptom, not a diagnosis.**

A. When a patient complains that he cannot sleep, your task is to identify the pattern and the probable cause of the sleep disturbance with a **thorough clinical sleep history.**

B. It is vital to also take a **targeted medical and psychiatric history** to assess for comorbidities.

HOT KEY The key to effective treatment of insomnia is taking a thorough sleep history.

---

   1. Get a picture of the patient's **24-hour sleep pattern.**
   a. What time does the patient get into bed?
   b. How long after getting into bed does the patient fall asleep?
   c. Once asleep, how long before the patient awakens?
   d. How many times does the patient awaken during the night?
   e. When does the patient get out of bed for the day?
   f. Does the patient nap? If so, when and for how long?

HOT KEY Many hospitalized patients nap so often during the day that their need for nighttime sleep is reduced, thereby producing "insomnia."

---

   2. Determine what, if any, **physical or mental symptoms** bother the patient when she is trying to sleep.

    a. Does the patient experience **pain, restlessness, or hot flashes?**

    b. Does the patient have **racing or intrusive thoughts or auditory hallucinations?**

    c. Is the patient hypervigilant or **fearful of the sleep environment?**

3. Determine **when the insomnia began** and if there is a history of previous sleep disorders.

    a. Has the patient had previous problems with sleep? What was happening in his life then? Was there a change in health? New medication? Stressful event?

    b. If so, how were the previous sleep disorders addressed?

4. Determine what **medications** (e.g., over-the-counter medications such as melatonin), **substances** (e.g., alcohol), or **herbal remedies** the patient has used to try to sleep.

5. If the patient is awake at night, determine what activities he engages in (e.g., stays in bed awake, eats, paces).

6. Assess the patient's **level of sleepiness during waking hours.** In addition to a thorough sleep history, it is important to evaluate the patient's functioning during waking hours to estimate the degree of excessive daytime sleepiness.

    a. Does the patient fall asleep during sedentary activities (e.g., reading, watching television, riding as a passenger in a vehicle)?

    b. Does the patient fall asleep at work? If so, does it happen while sitting or standing?

    c. Has the patient ever fallen asleep during a conversation?

    d. Has the patient ever fallen asleep while driving?

HOT KEY — Severe sleepiness is potentially lethal. Sleep bursts of only 10 seconds can occur in drowsy drivers, and 10 seconds at 55 miles per hour is 400 yards!

 TREATMENT

A. Transient or situational insomnia

1. If the insomnia is transient or appears to be situational and there are no contraindications, a **benzodiazepine** is an appropriate sedative-hypnotic to use for treatment. **The agent used should be determined based on the pattern of sleep disturbance.**

    a. If the patient's sole complaint is **initial insomnia,** a quick-onset, short half-life agent [e.g., zolpidem (Ambien), 5–10 mg, or zaleplon (Sonata), 5–10 mg] is ideal.

     b. For the patient with **middle or terminal insomnia** with situational anxiety use a benzodiazepine with a half-life of 6–8 hours or longer [e.g., temazepam (Restoril), 15–30 mg; diazepam (Valium), 5–10 mg; or clonazepam (Klonopin), 0.5–1.0 mg]. Medications such as zolpidem and triazolam are not appropriate choices because their 2–3 hour half-life means they will be metabolized by the time the patient needs help staying asleep. Moreover, these medications may cause more awakenings due to a within-night rebound phenomenon.

    2. In addition to treatment with a benzodiazepine, instruct the patient about proper **sleep hygiene** (Table 34-4).

B. Insomnia due to medication

    1. If it is possible to trace the onset of a sleep disturbance to the initiation of a medication, consider changing the dosing regimen to waking hours only (if possible) or switching to a non-activating medication.

    2. If a change in medication is not possible, administration of a sedative-hypnotic may be appropriate if the sleep disturbance is likely to continue if untreated.

C. Insomnia due to a medical or psychiatric illness

    1. If the sleep history has helped you to identify a correctable medical cause of the patient's sleep complaint (e.g., pain due to hip fracture), correct the problem. When medical illness produces insomnia, the sleep disturbance usually resolves when the medical illness is resolved.

    2. When a **psychiatric** illness produces insomnia, it is best to **treat the insomnia with a sedating medication in the same class that is being used to treat the illness.** If possible, treat the illness with a single agent that is sedating, thereby avoid-

---

TABLE 34-4. Guidelines for Good Sleep Hygiene

Ensure a quiet, comfortable sleep environment (consider earplugs if necessary)

Do not take any stimulants within 6 hours of bedtime

Reduce or eliminate caffeine; no caffeine within 6 hours of bedtime

Reduce nicotine

Keep a regular sleep schedule

Spend the last hour of the evening before bedtime relaxing

Reinforce waking hours with exposure to light early in the day

Exercise regularly, but not within 4 hours of bedtime

Limit activities in bed to sleep and sex

Restrict the amount of time spent in bed to the number of hours needed to sleep

ing polypharmacy. Following are some strategies for the treatment of psychiatric illnesses.

a. **Major depression.** Administer a sedating antidepressant (e.g., nefazodone, mirtazapine, imipramine) or add a low dose of a sedating antidepressant to the patient's current regimen (e.g., trazodone, 50–100 mg; amitriptyline, 5–20 mg; doxepin, 10–25 mg; mirtazapine, 7.5 mg).

b. **Mania.** Start with a mood stabilizer and then add a sedating antipsychotic (e.g., haloperidol, 5–10 mg), especially if the patient is psychotic, or a benzodiazepine (e.g., clonazepam, 0.5–1.0 mg; lorazepam, 1–2 mg).

c. **Psychosis.** Atypical antipsychotics may initially be activating, so add a low-potency typical antipsychotic (e.g., thioridazine, 50–100 mg) to facilitate sleep or use a high-potency antipsychotic as the primary treatment. Assess carefully for akathisia, and treat if necessary.

d. **Anxiety disorders.** Although the benzodiazepines are sedating and anxiolytic, they often are not the treatment of choice. Selective serotonin reuptake inhibitors (SSRIs) can be sedating or activating and are often the treatment of choice for anxiety disorders. Gabapentin (Neurontin) at up to 2400 mg/day in divided doses, may also be effective.

   (1) If insomnia complaints persist after administration of an SSRI, use low-dose benzodiazepines with a half-life of at least 6 hours (e.g., clonazepam, 0.5–1.0 mg; diazepam, 5–10 mg).

   (2) Do not use short-acting hypnotics (e.g., zolpidem) because the short half-life often exacerbates awakenings. Even alprazolam can worsen morning anxiety symptoms in sensitive patients.

e. **Substance abuse.** Medications play an important role in the withdrawal phase and the rehabilitation phase of treatment.

   (1) During acute withdrawal, sleep disturbances may be maximal, but are often ameliorated by the detoxification regimens (e.g., benzodiazepines for alcohol withdrawal).

   (2) Continued treatment of insomnia in the rehabilitation phase is often important to help maintain sobriety, but careful selection of agents is essential. Low-dose sedating tricyclic antidepressants (e.g., doxepin, 5–10 mg; trazodone, 50–100 mg) are often helpful. An assessment for underlying anxiety or mood disorder will also be important.

   (3) Although insomnia due to a psychiatric illness generally resolves when the illness is treated, people with a long history of drug or alcohol abuse may continue to have disrupted or unrefreshing sleep months or years after sobriety is achieved.

D. Psychophysiologic insomnia

1. Obsession with the inability to sleep manifests as **heightened levels of muscle tension and anxiety,** which directly interfere with sleep.

2. **Psychophysiologic insomnia is a diagnosis of exclusion,** and the presence of an underlying sleep disorder must be considered and, if present, treated before cognitive-behavioral therapy is attempted.

3. This persistent form of sleep disturbance usually resolves when a structured form of **cognitive-behavioral therapy and relaxation training** are applied over several weeks. Essentially, patients have to relearn how to let sleep happen.

VI FOLLOW-UP AND REFERRAL

A. If you suspect that a patient's sleep disturbance is due to a medical or psychiatric illness, it is best to have the treating physician reassess both the illness and the medications being used to treat the illness.

B. If a primary sleep disorder or psychophysiologic insomnia is suspected, a referral to a sleep disorder center is advised.

C. If the patient has transient insomnia and a short course of a sedative-hypnotic is used, the patient should be reassessed to ensure that the symptom of insomnia has resolved and that no untoward side effects (e.g., morning lethargy, confusion) are experienced. Once the medication is no longer needed, an appropriate tapering dose schedule should be planned so that rebound insomnia symptoms do not appear.

D. All patients will benefit from reminders about proper sleep hygiene (see Table 34-4).

References

Anonymous: Insomnia: Assessment and management in primary care. National Heart, Lung, and Blood Institute Working Group on Insomnia. *Am Fam Physician* 59(11):3029–3038, 1999.

Attarian HP: Helping patients who say they cannot sleep: Practical ways to evaluate and treat insomnia. *Postgrad Med* 107(3):127–130, 140–142, 2000.

Holbrook AM, Crowther R, Lotter A, et al: The diagnosis and management of insomnia in clinical practice: A practical evidence-based approach. *CMAJ* 162(2): 216–220, 2000.

Roth T: New trends in insomnia management. *J Psychopharmacol (Oxf)* 13(4 suppl 1):S37–40, 1999.

PART XII

SEXUALITY AND GENDER IDENTITY

35. Human Sexuality and Sexual Dysfunction

I **HUMAN SEXUALITY.** Human sexual behavior is a complex phenomenon that is influenced by **biologic, psychologic, and sociocultural factors.** Notions of normal versus deviant sexual behavior vary from culture to culture and from one historical period to another. Normal sexual development begins in infancy, leading to the formation of gender identity in the first years of life.

A. Infantile sexuality
1. As Freud noted nearly a century ago, children begin to handle and manipulate their genitals at a young age. By 18 months of age, most children begin genital self-stimulation and derive pleasure from the experience. They also become interested in the genitals of peers and adults.
2. Guilt-free genital exploration in infancy seems to lead to a more satisfactory and pleasurable adult sex life.

B. Human sexuality. There are three components that collectively define human sexuality: core gender identity, gender role identity, and sexual orientation.
1. **Core gender identity** is one's inner feeling of maleness or femaleness. It is thought to be fixed at approximately 18 months of age and is believed to be unchangeable. Core gender identity does not always correspond to a person's anatomic and biologic sex.
2. **Gender role identity** describes the set of personal attributes that a society identifies with males or females (e.g., passivity for women and aggressiveness for men in late Victorian Europe). Individuals can depart from socially constructed gender roles without having any conflict about their underlying core gender identity.

3. Sexual orientation describes an individual's dominant mode of sexual attraction (e.g., homosexual, heterosexual, bisexual).

HOT KEY

Conscious desire, not a particular sexual act, defines sexual orientation.

II **NORMAL SEXUAL RESPONSE.** Men and women experience **a four-phase response cycle** that involves increasing myotonia and vasoconstriction followed by decreasing myotonia and vasoconstriction.

A. Desire is the nonphysiologic, psychologic drive toward sexual activity. It includes sexual fantasies.

B. Excitement is the direct physical or psychologic stimulation that leads to a subjective experience of sexual pleasure. The physiologic consequences of excitement are:
  1. Penile tumescence
  2. Vaginal lubrication
  3. Erectile nipples
  4. Enlarged testicles and breasts
  5. Clitoral and labial engorgement
  6. Increased heart rate, respiration, and blood pressure

C. Orgasm is the phase during which sexual excitation reaches a peak. There is release of sexual tension and rhythmic movement of the perineal muscles and reproductive organs. Blood pressure rises and the heart rate increases to as high as 150–170 beats/min. On average, an orgasm lasts for 14 seconds.
  1. In men, orgasm consists of ejaculation and four to five spasms of the urethra and prostate.
  2. In women, orgasm involves involuntary contractions of the lower vagina and uterus.

D. Resolution is the period after orgasm during which the body slowly returns to a nonstimulated state.

HOT KEY

Before renewed sexual activity, men have a refractory period ranging from several minutes to several hours during which they need to be "recharged." Women usually do not have a refractory period.

III **SEXUAL DYSFUNCTION**

A. Introduction
  1. Any disturbance in the sexual response cycle, pain, or loss of

pleasure during sexual intercourse, or loss in desire for sexual pleasure is described as sexual dysfunction.

2. It is difficult to obtain prevalence rates for sexual dysfunction because it can be associated with psychiatric syndromes, physiologic influences, and pharmacologic influences.

3. It is more common for patients to present with new onset of dysfunction rather than a lifelong problem. Occasionally, a patient will report dysfunction only with one particular partner.

B. Clinical manifestations of sexual dysfunction (Table 35-1) include:

1. Hypoactive sexual desire
2. Avoidance of or aversion to sexual activities
3. Difficulty in orgasmic capacity
4. Pain during sexual intercourse

C. Causes of sexual dysfunction

1. Sexual dysfunction can be related to a **medical illness** (e.g., 20%–50% of men with erectile disorder have an organic basis for the disorder). Medical illnesses implicated in sexual dysfunction include:
   a. Diabetes mellitus
   b. Hypothyroidism
   c. Multiple sclerosis
   d. Peripheral neuropathy due to any cause (e.g., alcoholism)
   e. Tabes dorsalis

TABLE 35-1. Clinical Manifestations of Common Sexual Dysfunctions

Dysfunction	Clinical Manifestations
Female sexual arousal disorder	Inability to attain or maintain an adequate lubrication and swelling response of sexual excitement during sexual activity
Male erectile disorder	Inability to attain or maintain an erection
Premature ejaculation	Early or immediate ejaculation (often prior to penetration) that precludes a satisfying sexual encounter for both partners
Dyspareunia	Persistent genital pain associated with sexual activity (in men or women)
Vaginismus	Involuntary spasm of the muscles of the outer third of the vagina that interferes with sexual activity

2. **Substance abuse and medications** are frequent causes of sexual dysfunction, especially in men. Commonly prescribed medications that may cause dysfunction include:
   a. Antiparkinsonian agents (e.g., levodopa)
   b. Propranolol
   c. Digoxin
   d. Clonidine
   e. Hydrochlorothiazide
   f. Spironolactone
   g. Haloperidol
   h. Risperidone
   i. Fluphenazine
   j. Sertraline
   k. Paroxetine
   l. Fluoxetine
   m. Lithium

> **HOT KEY**
>
> Drug abuse is very common and often leads to sexual dysfunction (e.g., alcohol increases sexual drive but decreases sexual performance).

3. **Psychiatric syndromes** (e.g., depression) are frequently associated with a loss of sexual desire, in which case the primary psychiatric disorder must be treated first.
D. Approach to the patient

> **HOT KEY**
>
> Clinicians working with patients who present problems related to sexuality need to be vigilant to convey an accepting, nonjudgmental attitude.

1. Patients are often hesitant to broach the topic of sexual dysfunction, so be sure to **ask explicitly about sexual functioning** as part of the routine assessment.
2. If the patient identifies sexual dysfunction as a problem, **subsequent questions** should focus on:
   a. Specific symptoms (e.g., loss of desire, loss of ability to participate sexually, pain)
   b. When the symptoms began and with what partner
   c. Any concurrent medications and medical problems
   d. Any psychiatric symptoms or medications

    e. Use of alcohol and other substances

    f. Attempts the patient has made to enhance sexual activity

E. Treatment

HOT KEY

If the patient is male, inquire about early-morning erections. If the patient does awake with an erection, then the cause is most likely psychologic, not organic.

---

1. First **identify or rule out organic causes** of sexual dysfunction.
   a. If an organic cause is identified, appropriate intervention should be initiated. Consider referring the patient to an internist, urologist, or gynecologist as appropriate.
   b. If organic causes are ruled out, proceed with psychologic treatment.

HOT KEY

Sildenafil citrate (Viagra) is being used as a remedy for erectile dysfunction; however, it requires the presence of sexual desire. Viagra is not effective in people with loss of sexual desire. It is contraindicated in patients taking nitrate-containing medications (e.g., nitroglycerin).

---

2. **Psychologic treatment** for sexual dysfunction ranges from **sex therapy with the couple** to **behavioral or analytically oriented individual therapy.**
   a. Behavior therapy uses techniques to enhance the sexual response of one or both partners. For example, in the case of vaginismus, a woman is advised to dilate her vaginal opening with her fingers or a dilation device before intercourse.
   b. Analytically oriented individual therapy may be appropriate, for example, in the treatment of someone with sexual aversion disorder, whose problem with sexual contact is rooted in a fear of intimacy.
   c. Sex therapy with the couple draws upon many modalities—behavior modification, relaxation exercises, and couples dynamic therapy—to define and then correct the sexual conflict. For instance, "homework" assignments of having foreplay without the expectation of intercourse to reduce performance anxiety and to foster a desire to explore each other's bodies.

References

Kafka MP: Hypersexual desire in males. *Arch Sex Behav* 26(5):505–526, 1997.

O'Donohue W, Dopke CA, Swingen DN: Psychotherapy for female sexual dysfunction: A review. *Clin Psychol Rev* 17(5):537–566, 1997.

Robbins M: Nature, nurture and core gender identity. *J Am Psychoanal Assoc* 44(suppl):93–117, 1996.

36. Paraphilias

I INTRODUCTION

A. **Definition.** A paraphilia is a recurrent **sexual behavior, fantasy,** or **strong urge** that is:
   1. **Distressing** to the individual or to others;
   2. **Focused on humiliation** (of oneself or others), on children, on nonconsenting adults, or on nonhuman objects.

B. **Types**
   1. **Pedophilia:** recurrent sexual fantasies, urges, or sexual activity involving prepubescent children.
   2. **Fetishism:** recurrent sexually arousing fantasies, urges, or behavior involving the use of nonliving objects (e.g., women's shoes).
   3. **Exhibitionism:** recurrent sexually arousing fantasies, urges, or behavior involving the exposure of one's genitals to an unsuspecting stranger.
   4. **Voyeurism:** recurrent preoccupation with people who are naked or involved in sexual activity.
   5. **Sadomasochism:** recurrent preoccupation with sexual urges or actions involving oneself or a sexual partner being humiliated, beaten, bound, or made to suffer.
   6. **Frotteurism:** recurrent fantasies or behavior involving anonymous rubbing of one's genitals against strangers in public, leading to orgasm.

C. **Incidence**
   1. **Pedophilia is the most common paraphilia.** In some studies it is estimated that as many as 20% of children have been molested by adults before they reach 18 years of age. Most pedophiles are heterosexual males who are either part of the family or are closely involved with the families of the children they molest.
   2. **Onset** of most paraphilias, including pedophilia, **is prior to adulthood.**
   3. Paraphilias are significantly **more common in men.**

D. **Prognosis is poor.** Only long-term therapy is shown to be of some benefit. In pedophilia, medications have been shown to be of some value.

II CLINICAL MANIFESTATIONS

A. Manifestation of the paraphilias is often elusive because:
   1. People **hide their symptoms.**

2. People **might not desire a change in their sexual behavior** and are unwilling to undergo treatment.

B. People **may present for treatment only after they have gotten into legal trouble** as a consequence of their sexual behavior.

C. Although distressing, **people may feel that their sexual behavior is not the main problem,** and may instead focus on other aspects of their relationship troubles.

D. Patients may have multiple paraphilias.

III CAUSES

A. Psychoanalytic theory is the only school of thought available that attempts to describe the cause of paraphilias.

B. The current understanding is that **the patient turns toward the unusual methods of sexual gratification to manage some form of anxiety** associated with a normal method of sexual gratification.

 An adult patient with pedophilia was himself molested as a child. The adult in this case is thought to be attempting to manage his trauma by identifying with the aggressor.

IV APPROACH TO THE PATIENT

A. Patients would rarely seek treatment for paraphilias voluntarily. Therefore, **the clinician should ask explicit questions about sexual function** (not necessarily paraphilias), and if the patient is evasive or defensive, keep in mind that one reason he might be so is because of a paraphilia.

B. The clinician should take a **nonjudgmental approach** to help the patient realize that the goal is to help.

 HOT KEY Just because a patient is defensive or reluctant to talk about his sexual life does not mean that he has a paraphilia. Usually a patient will divulge this information only if he has a long-term relationship with his physician.

V TREATMENT tends to be challenging because in many instances the patient **does not seek treatment voluntarily** and paraphilias **are often refractory to treatment.**

A. **Insight-oriented psychotherapy** is the most common approach.

B. **Medications** have been used in conjunction with psychotherapy for treatment of paraphilias.

1. Anti-androgens [e.g., medroxyprogesterone acetate (Depo-Provera)] have been used, especially in hypersexual para-philiacs, resulting in some decrease in the sexual behavior.
2. Selective serotonin reuptake inhibitors (SSRIs) have also been used to treat obsessive sexual symptoms and sexual "addictions."

C. **Aversion therapy**—a form of punishment (such as electric shock) paired with images of the sexual behavior—has been used with limited success.

 FOLLOW-UP. Patients with pedophilia **require careful follow-up and referral to ensure safety of children.**

HOT KEY

> Physicians are mandated to report any sexual abuse of children to the appropriate state child protection services. In addition, if a patient appears to be planning a sexual assault or rape in the context of a paraphilia, the physician has a legal and ethical responsibility to report this to the intended victim.

References
Gayford JJ: Paraphilias: A review of the literature. *Med Sci Law* 37(4):303–315, 1997.
de Silva WP: ABC of sexual health. Sexual variations. *BMJ* 318(7184):654–656, 1999.
Zonana HV, Norko MA: Sexual predators. *Psych Clin North Am* 22(1):109–127, vii, 1999.

37. Gender Identity Disorder

I **INTRODUCTION.** To understand gender identity disorder, one must first have a clear understanding of core gender identity (see Chapter 35).

A. Definition. The presence of a **strong and persistent transgender identification** and **a persistent discomfort about one's biologic sex** indicates a gender identity disorder. There must be significant distress or impairment in functioning, and there is no physical intersex condition.

B. Incidence. Very little data are available as to the prevalence of this disorder, although **men and boys tend to be more commonly affected.**

II **CLINICAL MANIFESTATIONS**

A. Manifestations in children
1. In boys, common presentations of gender identity disorder include the **desire to grow up to be a woman** and **repulsion toward their genitals.**
2. In girls, common presentations include **a preference for only male playmates** and **an expressed preference to be a boy.**

B. Manifestations in adolescents and adults
1. Unlike children, adolescents and adults with gender identity disorder are able to state their desires more clearly and **want to acquire the sexual characteristics of the opposite sex.** Statements like "I feel like a woman trapped in a male body" are common.
2. Patients may request hormonal treatment and surgical procedures to alter their physical appearance. The term **transsexual** is applied to people who undergo such treatment. There are male-to-female transsexuals and female-to-male transsexuals.

HOT KEY A patient with a core gender identity different from his or her biologic gender is referred to as a **transgender** person. Occasionally, transgender patients become **transsexual** by undergoing treatments to alter their physical appearance.

C. Sexual orientation is independent of core gender identity—patients with gender identity disorder could be attracted to either males or females or both even if they were male-to-female transsexuals.

III CAUSES

A. The causes of gender identity disorder are unclear.
B. Some data available from sex assignment of children born with ambiguous genitalia indicate that irrespective of the biologic sex of the child, in most cases the child's core gender identity corresponds to his or her biologic gender.

IV DIFFERENTIAL DIAGNOSIS.
In certain cultures there is confusion between sexual orientation and core gender identity. It is sometimes thought that if one is attracted to a same-sex partner, one wishes to be a member of the opposite sex. Occasionally, patients may present with confusion about this, but they usually conclude over time that, while their sexual preference is homosexual, they do not have real conflict over their core gender identity.

V APPROACH TO THE PATIENT

A. **The clinician should probably not try to change a child's core gender identity.** Core gender identity is formed by the age of approximately 18 months and is unchangeable later in life. Some clinicians have attempted to help children change their gender identity, and even though some of them have reported "success," there are no studies demonstrating a true core gender identity change.
B. The psychiatrist should ask the patient how he or she would like to be addressed and should respect the patient's preference. Some patients prefer to use a gender-neutral name, while others have a strong preference to be addressed as "he" or "she" or "Mr." or "Ms.," despite outward appearances.

VI TREATMENT

A. **Psychoanalytic psychotherapy** is helpful to patients of any age who have feelings of depression and anxiety associated with gender identity disorder.
B. For adults who are committed to transitioning to the other sex, there are **three stages** of treatment a patient undergoes to achieve a successful transsexual transition: **psychotherapy, hormone therapy,** and **sex-reassignment surgery.**
   1. **Psychotherapy** can be invaluable in helping pre- and post-operative transsexuals cope with the emotions involved in contemplating or adjusting to such a significant life change.

2. **Hormone therapy** involves **testosterone** for female-to-male transsexual patients and **estradiol** and **progesterone** for male-to-female transsexual patients. After several months of hormone treatment, the patient's body shape begins to change. Men who are taking hormones find their breasts enlarged and fat redistributed. Women taking testosterone become amenorrheic and have a deeper voice, clitoral enlargement, and also some increase in facial hair. In addition, because of the hormone therapy, patients need to be monitored by a physician for **hypertension, hepatic dysfunction, thromboembolic phenomena, and hyperglycemia,** which are all potential side effects of taking hormones.

3. In the United States, prior to undergoing sex reassignment, patients are required by consensus to undergo psychotherapy and hormone treatments and to live for a period of time as a transgender person. Many such patients already are doing so, though if the patient opts to go abroad for surgery there are no such requirements.

VII FOLLOW-UP

A. The majority of patients who have undergone sex-reassignment surgery report satisfactory sex after surgery.

B. **Ongoing psychotherapy is very beneficial** to all transsexual patients. Living a life as a transsexual means relating to friends, family, and lovers differently. In addition, transsexual patients often face the ongoing stressors of discrimination and maltreatment.

HOT KEY

It is important to note that many transgender patients elect not to have complete sex-reassignment surgery.

References

Cohen-Kettenis PT, Gooren LJ: Transsexualism: A review of etiology, diagnosis and treatment. *J Psychosom Res* 46(4):315–333, 1999.

Midence K, Hargreaves I: Psychosocial adjustment in male-to-female transsexuals: An overview of the research evidence. *J Psychol* 131(6):602–614, 1997.

PART XIII

CHILD AND ADOLESCENT PSYCHIATRY

38. Development

I DEVELOPMENT

A. Development is the **orderly and cumulative process of change and maturation across a person's life span** (i.e., from conception to death).

> **HOT KEY**
>
> An individual's development is the result of the interplay of genetic, biological, experiential, and environmental factors.

B. Development generally occurs in small steps that progress from basic to more complex. Early stage models of development (Table 38-1) depicted development as a progression of concrete, sequential, unidirectional stages. Today, researchers have demonstrated that while it does follow a sequence of phases, development is flexible, fluid, multidirectional, and interrelated to the developmental progression of other abilities.

C. There are **sensitive periods** during which humans are optimally primed by biological and genetic predispositions to make certain developmental changes.

1. Genes and their biological expression work together to create an environment of sensitivity for the developmental change to occur (e.g., primary language acquisition). These sensitive periods provide a window for full development that ultimately closes (or becomes significantly more limited) if sufficient stimulation is not provided. For example, genes create the brain structures that are primed to acquire language when given language input by caregivers in the environment.

2. The environment provides influence through both stimulation and stressors.

a. When the environmental stimulation is **normal,** the individual achieves steps toward more advanced development. For example, babies babble and respond when others speak or babble in return; the parents help shape the babbling into recognizable words.

b. **Overstimulation** (e.g., a traumatic first day of school negatively impacting language fluency) or **understimulation** (e.g., lack of language input from caregivers) may interfere with development. **Premature stimulation** may also interfere with development (e.g., sexual molestation may negatively impact later sexual development).

c. **Intervention** for developmental deviations and insults is **commonly successful,** but requires intensive efforts to achieve adequate but occasionally suboptimal development. For example, speech and language therapy several times per week may help with delays and articulation difficulties, but the child may still have reading and academic problems later in life.

HOT

KEY

All individuals go through similar developmental changes, but each does so in a unique manner.

▌ II ▐ THE DEVELOPMENTAL PERSPECTIVE

A. The **developmental model** of conceptualizing patient difficulties is very **different than the traditional medical model.**

   1. The traditional medical model is linear: **Diagnosis** is based on **symptoms,** which lead to a prescribed **treatment.**

   2. The developmental model relies on the **normal progression of child and adolescent development** as a **backdrop against which to assess difficulties** in a patient.

B. The concept of a **developmental age** is important to the developmental model.

   1. The range of development normally associated with the child's chronological age creates an expected range of normal functioning.

   2. This expected range sets a standard for evaluating the difficulties experienced by the patient (i.e., chronological age plus or minus one year is generally considered within normal limits).

C. Using a developmental perspective, when a child or adolescent is brought in for evaluation of his or her difficulties, the provider notes all of the following in assessing the degree to which symptoms are impeding normal functioning.

1. The child's current symptoms (i.e., physical, emotional, behavioral)
2. The normality of the difficulties for that developmental age (e.g., babbling is normal in a 1-year-old child but not in a 5-year-old)
3. How previous developmental insults, disturbances, or pervasive or specific delays may be contributing to the current symptoms. For example, frequent ear infections or injury to the dominant brain hemisphere may impact language development later in life.
4. The child's reaction to the difficulties and the resiliency of the child. For example, articulation difficulties may affect the child's self-esteem.
5. Ways in which the difficulties may be impacting functioning in the home, school, and community. For example, a child with a language disorder may suffer from social isolation.
6. Caregiver interactions with the child. For example, the parent may feel guilty about the child's difficulties and, as a result, overindulge or protect him.
7. Broader systemic issues. For example, because of inadequate medical insurance, school district funding, or family finances, the child may not have access to optimal treatment.
8. It is important that the clinician understand the symptoms and problems from the child's perspective.

References

MacWhinney B: Models of the emergence of language. *Annu Rev Psychol* 49:199–227, 1998.

Ollendick TH, Vasey MW: Developmental theory and the practice of clinical psychology. *J Clin Child Psychol* 28(4):457–466, 1999.

TABLE 38-1 Stage Models of Development

Age	Freud's Psychosexual Stages and Theory of the Child's Sensory Organization	Erikson's Psychosocial Stages and Developmental Tasks of the Stages	Piaget's Cognitive Development Stages and Description of Changes in Cognitive Capacities
Birth to 1 year	Oral (0–18 months)—Experience is based on pleasures from the mouth region.	Trust vs. mistrust (0–18 months)—Infant learns to trust caregivers to be responsive to his or her physical and emotional needs.	Sensorimotor (0–24 months)—Infant progresses from simple reflexes and instinctual actions to early symbolic thought. Sensory experiences and physical actions become organized into a constructed view of the world.
1 to 2 years	Anal (18–36 months)—Experience is based on pleasures from elimination.	Autonomy vs. shame and doubt (12–24 months)—Child's drive for independence and self-sufficiency emerge. Ability to follow social rules develops. If sense of competency is not achieved, shame and self-doubt predominate.	
3 to 5 years	Phallic (3–6 years)—Experience is based on pleasures from and awareness of genitals. Oedipus conflicts develop in response to genital awakening.	Initiative vs. guilt (3–5 years)—Increased social experience allows for greater control over purposeful behavior. Ability to evaluate intentions and behaviors develops. Guilty feelings	Pre-Operational (2–7 years)—Child is able to develop a mental construction of the world with language and images, reflecting the

	may arise if child is irresponsible and punitively corrected.	increased capacity for symbolic thinking. Planning and problem-solving go beyond connections between sensory information and physical actions. Basic conceptual development emerges.
6 to 12 years	Latency (6 years to puberty)—Child represses all focus on sexuality; energy is channeled into mastery of social and intellectual skills.	Industry vs. inferiority (6 years to puberty)—Child has enthusiasm about creation, imagination, mastery of information, and problem-solving ability. Possibly struggles with a lack of success, and feelings of incompetence may develop.	Concrete operations (7–11 years)—The ability to use reasoning to process information logically, systematically, and to organize and classify objects and information emerges.
13 to Young adulthood	Genital (puberty to adulthood)—Individual has period of sexual reawakening. Focus is on finding a partner outside the family for sexual gratification and adult relations.	Identity vs. identity confusion (10–20 years)—Individuals find and establish who they are, what their interests and goals are in life. Experimentation with lifestyles and roles occurs.	Formal operations (11–15 years)—Adolescents become capable of abstract thought, able to test hypotheses, and to plan and anticipate consequences. Idealistic thinking emerges.

(continued)

TABLE 38-1 Stage Models of Development (Continued)			
Age	Freud's Psychosexual Stages and Theory of the Child's Sensory Organization	Erikson's Psychosocial Stages and Developmental Tasks of the Stages	Piaget's Cognitive Development Stages and Description of Changes in Cognitive Capacities
20 to 40 years		Intimacy vs. isolation (Early adulthood)—Young adults face the task of forming intimate relationships; find and redefine oneself through the relationship with a partner.	
40 to 60 years		Generativity vs. stagnation (Middle adulthood)—Adult is established in life's work; focus is shifted to helping the younger generation lead useful lives.	
60+ years		Integrity vs. despair (Late adulthood)—Adult reflects upon life, evaluates life's work, and evaluates self in those retrospective reflections.	

39. Developmental Disorders

I. PERVASIVE DEVELOPMENTAL DISORDERS (PDDs)

A. **Introduction.** The spectrum of pervasive developmental disorders includes autistic disorder, Asperger's disorder, Rett's disorder, childhood disintegrative disorder, and pervasive developmental disorder not otherwise specified (PDD NOS). These disorders are **severe, present early in life,** and **affect children's development in multiple spheres** (hence the term "pervasive").

B. **Clinical manifestations of pervasive developmental disorders**

1. **Autistic disorder (autism)** has a prevalence of approximately 1 in 1000. Autistic disorder occurs more commonly in boys, but affected girls tend to have more severe mental retardation. Autistic disorder is the best characterized of the disorders in this class. The affected individual shows impairment in three major areas.

   a. **Reciprocal social interaction.** Interest in and ability to interact with others appropriately is impaired.

   b. **Communication.** Verbal and nonverbal communication are not used in an age-appropriate or communicative manner. Communication difficulties may also manifest as a lack of imaginative play.

   c. **Restricted repertoire of behaviors, interests,** and **activities.** This may include stereotyped movements, preoccupations, or ritualized behaviors.

2. **Asperger's disorder** is similar to autism except that the clinically significant delays in language and cognitive development that are found in autism are not found in Asperger's disorder. Unusual circumscribed interests are often found, and motor deficits may be prominent. This disorder is more common in males than females.

3. **Rett's disorder** is characterized by normal development for at least 5 months with subsequent regression. Features include deceleration of head growth, loss of purposeful hand movements replaced by characteristic hand-wringing motions, mental retardation, lack of social interest, and impairments in coordination and language. Rett's disorder has been seen only in females.

4. **Childhood disintegrative disorder** is marked by significant regression that occurs following normal development up to at least 2 years of age. This regression occurs in at least two of the following areas: language, social skills, bowel or blad-

der control, play, or motor skills, and two of the three symptom clusters of autism.

5. **PDD NOS** is the **most common diagnosis** for children with PDD spectrum disorders. This is a subthreshold diagnosis for those who possess some of the features of the other pervasive developmental disorders, but do not meet specific criteria for any of them.

C. **Etiology of pervasive developmental disorders**
   1. **Neurobiological factors** appear to play a critical role in the pathogenesis of pervasive developmental disorders.
      a. Autism may be associated with **medical conditions,** such as **fragile X syndrome** or **tuberous sclerosis.**
      b. The differential sex ratios in Rett's disorder and Asperger's disorder and the increased familial risk in autistic disorder and Asperger's disorder suggest **genetic contributions,** most likely according to a **polygenic model.**
      c. **Structural brain abnormalities** are associated with pervasive developmental disorders. There is an association of autism with tuberous sclerosis, findings of macrocephaly in one third of children with PDD, enlargement of certain cortical areas in men with autism, and hypoplasia of the cerebellum.
      d. **Soft neurologic signs** or abnormal electroencephalograms (EEGs) may be seen even without seizure disorder.
      e. Some patients with autism have **elevated peripheral serotonin** levels with a possible disturbance in uptake regulation.
   2. **Current theories** about the nature of the **critical deficit** in PDD spectrum disorders include:
      a. **Central coherence theory,** which proposes that affected individuals have difficulty seeing the "big picture," instead focusing on components.
      b. **Executive or frontal lobe functioning theory,** which posits a deficit in planfulness and appreciation of long-term consequences.
      c. **Theory of the Mind,** which proposes that pervasive developmental disorders are caused by a difficulty in thinking about others' thoughts. This difficulty results in a lack of understanding that others operate with intentions built upon beliefs.
      d. **Early disturbances of social meaning theory,** which posits a disturbance in social interest, mediated by very specific parts of the brain.

D. **Differential diagnosis and comorbid conditions**
   1. **Differential diagnosis** includes:
      a. Mental retardation

b. Deafness in infants and toddlers
c. Language disorders
d. Selective mutism
e. Reactive attachment disorder
f. Obsessive–compulsive disorder
g. Schizophrenia
h. Schizoid personality disorder
2. Comorbid conditions
a. Mental retardation (see II) is a common finding with all of the pervasive developmental disorders except Asperger's disorder.

HOT KEY

Seventy-five percent of children with autism also have mental retardation.

b. Seizure disorders

HOT KEY

Up to 30% of children with pervasive developmental disorders may have seizure disorders.

c. Obsessive-compulsive behaviors
d. Attention-deficit/hyperactivity disorder (ADHD) symptoms
e. Mood disorders
f. Stereotyped movements
g. Aggressivity
h. Self-injurious behavior
i. Psychotic symptoms
E. Approach to the patient. Work-up should be guided by history and clinical findings and should include:
1. A developmental and medical history
2. A complete physical examination, including complete blood cell count, urinalysis, and liver function tests
3. Psychological testing to assess the child's cognitive profile, academic functioning, speech and language functioning, adaptive functioning, and strengths and weaknesses
4. A diagnostic examination with observation in various settings including interaction with parents, interaction with strangers, during play, and while performing structured tasks. Diagnostic instruments may be helpful.

5. A psychiatric evaluation should be performed if there is reason to suspect comorbid psychiatric conditions.
6. For very young children, a **hearing test** or test of auditory evoked potentials may be indicated to rule out deafness as a cause of communication difficulties.
7. A **neurologic evaluation** may be indicated, especially if there is concern about seizure disorder.
8. A **genetics referral** may be warranted if family history or dysmorphic features are present.

F. **Treatment and prognosis**
1. **Intense, early intervention** appears to be critical for positive outcome. This may include services such as speech and occupational therapy, special education, behavior therapy, and support in acquiring social and self-help skills.
2. However, there is **no proven treatment** for the deficits underlying PDD spectrum disorders. Associated psychiatric issues may require psychopharmacologic management if they interfere with the patient's ability to remain safe, to learn, or to be adequately cared for. This treatment is directed at symptoms only. **Antipsychotics, antidepressants, and mood stabilizers are often used.**
3. One third of patients with autism may live partially independent lives as adults. Only a very small minority will lead fully independent lives. The degree of language impairment and mental retardation strongly predict outcome.

II MENTAL RETARDATION

A. **Overview.** Mental retardation is an Axis II condition marked by **significantly subaverage intelligence quotient (IQ)** with **impairment of adaptive functioning.** The prevalence rate is roughly 1%. Mental retardation is characterized as follows:
   Mild (IQ level 50–55 to approximately 70)
   Moderate (IQ level 35–40 to 50–55)
   Severe (IQ level 20–25 to 35–40)
   Profound (IQ level below 20 or 25)
B. **Etiology.** Mental retardation represents the final common pathway of a heterogeneous group of factors. **Causation is multifactorial.** In 30% of cases, no identifiable cause is found. Socioeconomic status is more strongly associated with mild than with more severe forms of mental retardation, which appear to be more strongly related to organic causes.
1. **Organic factors** include congenital syndromes (e.g., metabolic illnesses, Down syndrome, fetal alcohol syndrome), pregnancy-related problems (e.g., maternal infections or asphyxia with consequent cerebral palsy and mental retardation), acquired insults (e.g., lead ingestion or head trauma), and others.

    2. Polygenic influences. Fifty percent of the variability in IQ appears to be genetically mediated through polygenic mechanisms.

    3. Sociocultural factors include an inadequately stimulating environment and inadequate schooling.

C. Comorbid conditions are three to four times greater in children with mental retardation. This association is strongest for children with lower levels of IQ. Comorbid conditions include:

    1. ADHD

    2. Pervasive developmental disorders

    3. Mood disorders

    4. Aggression

    5. Stereotypies

    6. Self-injurious behavior

III LEARNING DISORDERS are diagnosed when **academic performance does not measure up to ability.**

A. Epidemiology. Five percent of children in the United States have been diagnosed with learning disorders, including reading disorder, mathematics disorder, and disorder of written expression.

B. Approach to the patient. Psychoeducational testing and appropriate special educational supports are indicated.

C. Comorbid conditions. ADHD, behavioral disorders, mood disorders, communication disorders, or other learning disorders may be comorbid and should be a focus of treatment (see Chapters 41 and 42).

IV COMMUNICATION DISORDERS include expressive language disorder, mixed expressive-receptive language disorder, phonologic disorder, and stuttering.

References

Toppelberg CO, Shapiro T: Language disorders: A 10-year research update review. *J Am Acad Child Adolesc Psychiatry* 39(2):143–152, 2000.

Volkmar F, et al: Practice parameters for the assessment and treatment of children, adolescents, and adults with autism and other pervasive developmental disorders. *J Am Acad Child Adolesc Psychiatry* 38(suppl)12:325–545, 1999.

40. Anxiety and Tic Disorders in Childhood and Adolescence

❚ ANXIETY DISORDERS

A. Introduction

1. **Prevalence.** Anxiety disorders may be the **most prevalent** psychiatric disorders of childhood. **Prevalence increases through adolescence.**

2. **Types.** Anxiety disorders that present in children include:
   a. **separation anxiety disorder**
   b. **selective mutism**
   c. **anxiety disorders that are also seen in adulthood** (e.g., specific and social phobias, panic disorder, generalized anxiety disorder, obsessive–compulsive disorder, post-traumatic stress disorder)

HOT KEY

Children with anxiety disorders are at greatly increased risk of developing other anxiety disorders in childhood and adolescence.

3. While the specific anxiety disorder diagnosed in a child may change over time, children with anxiety disorders tend to **remain within the spectrum of anxiety and depressive disorders.**

4. **Temperament** and **parental behaviors** appear to **play significant roles,** especially regarding autonomy, attachment, and reinforcement of fears.

5. **Common comorbid conditions** include:
   a. Depressive disorders (see Chapter 41)
   b. Disruptive behavior disorders and attention-deficit hyperactivity disorder (ADHD) (see Chapter 42).

6. For children and adolescents who do not display disruptive behaviors, anxiety disorders may go unrecognized and untreated.

HOT KEY

Parents tend to report fewer anxiety symptoms for their children than children report for themselves. Therefore, it is important to include the child's self-report in the assessment.

B. General approach to the patient and treatment of anxiety disorders

   1. Assessment should include developmental history (with a focus on temperament and attachment), school, family, and medical history (including medications and illnesses which may mimic anxiety) (see Chapter 18 V D, E, F).

   2. Cognitive behavioral and **behavioral treatments** have been widely and effectively used to treat these disorders.

   3. Other approaches

   a. Psychoeducation, relaxation training, family, group, and psychodynamically oriented therapies have been effective. Helping parents to understand their child's difficulties and guiding parents in ways in which to respond can be useful.

   b. Medication can be useful but should play only an **adjunctive role.** Medications used for anxiety disorders include tricyclic antidepressants, selective serotonin reuptake inhibitors (SSRIs), and benzodiazepines for short-term use. β-Blockers, monoamine oxidase inhibitors (MAOIs), antihistamines, and buspirone are also used.

C. Specific types of anxiety disorders

   1. Separation anxiety disorder

   a. Overview. This disorder involves excessive anxiety upon separation from home or attachment figures, lasting at least 4 weeks, to a degree that is impairing and greater than developmentally expected. Prevalence is around 4%. Peak incidence is at 11 years of age. Separation anxiety disorder may be associated with somatic complaints related to separating from parents. It may develop following a major stressor. School phobia, panic disorder with agoraphobia, and depressive disorders may ensue. Separation anxiety disorders cluster in families—parents may have panic disorder, agoraphobia, or depression.

   b. Differential diagnosis includes developmentally normal separation anxiety, simple truancy, panic disorder, generalized anxiety disorder, school phobia, and depressive disorders.

   c. Treatment

   (1) The child needs to separate from the parent and discover that the associated fears are unfounded. It is important to **educate the parents** about this so that their own anxieties do not interfere with the child's ability to separate.

   (2) Medications. Imipramine (Tofranil) at doses of 3–5 mg/kg/day, alprazolam (Xanax) (up to 1 mg/day), diphenhydramine (Benadryl), or buspirone (BuSpar) may be helpful. Baseline and follow-up electrocardiograms must be checked when administering tricyclic antidepressants, such as imipramine.

2. Selective mutism

  a. Overview. This disorder is characterized by the patient's failure to speak in certain social situations, despite ability to speak in others. It lasts at least one month, to a degree that causes impairment. It generally presents before 5 years of age. Prevalence is less than 1%. The disorder is more common in girls than in boys. Speech and language disorders may be comorbid, but are not severe enough to explain the lack of speech.

  b. Differential diagnosis includes communication disorders, lack of knowledge of the language, social phobia, pervasive developmental disorder (PDD) spectrum disorders, and psychotic disorders.

  c. Treatment

   (1) Behavioral modification approaches are often used.

   (2) Medications. Paroxetine (Paxil) as well as α-agonists such as guanfacine (Tenex) or clonidine (Catapres) may be helpful (see Chapter 42 I).

3. Specific and social phobias

  a. Overview—DSM-IV criteria are the same as for adults (see Chapter 19 II) except for the stipulation that symptoms must be present for more than 6 months. This helps prevent the misdiagnosis of developmentally normal fears as phobias. The criteria do not require that children recognize the excessive nature of their fears. DSM-IV allows that children may express their anxiety through crying, tantrums, clinging, or "freezing." The nature of phobias is informed by the developmental level. Prevalence estimates for simple phobia are relatively high, ranging from 2%–9%.

  b. Differential diagnosis. Developmentally normal fears should be considered first. Other anxiety disorders and psychotic disorders should also be considered. Withdrawn behavior associated with depressive disorders may present similarly to phobias. School avoidance may evolve into school phobia.

  c. Treatment

   (1) Behavioral therapies, including **systematic desensitization** and prolonged exposure, are particularly useful in the treatment of phobias.

   (2) Medications. Benzodiazepines may be useful for severe symptoms. Imipramine (Tofranil) may be useful for school phobia. The β-blocker propranolol (Inderal) may be useful for stage fright. However, a baseline electrocardiogram should be performed and blood pressures need to be followed. This medication is contraindicated in patients with asthma, diabetes, and heart block.

HOT

 Onset of social phobia is usually after 10 years of age and incidence increases markedly with age.

KEY

---

4. **Panic disorder**
   a. **Overview.** Panic attacks tend to be connected with other anxiety disorders in childhood. Panic disorder occurs more frequently in adolescents than children. Adolescents possess the cognitive capacity to worry about losing control. In adolescents, the presentation of panic disorder is similar to that in adults. DSM-IV criteria are the same as for adults (see Chapter 18 II B 1).
   b. **Differential diagnosis** of panic disorder in children is the same as for adults (see Chapter 18 V).
   c. **Treatment**
      (1) Combinations of psychotherapy and medication management may be particularly useful for adolescents.
      (2) Psychotherapy may focus on underlying conflicts.
      (3) Medications—tricyclic antidepressants such as imipramine (Tofranil) and desipramine (Norpramin), as well as benzodiazepines may be useful (see C 1 c (2)).
5. **Generalized anxiety disorder**
   a. **Overview.** DSM-IV criteria are the same as for adults except that only one symptom of tension and vigilance is required for diagnosis in children, as opposed to three for adults. Prevalence is around 3%. This disorder tends to present during the later school-age years. An equal male to female ratio of generalized anxiety disorder is seen until adolescence, when girls outnumber boys 6 to 1.
   b. **Differential diagnosis** includes the other anxiety disorders, effects of drugs or medications, or underlying medical problems (see Chapter 17 V D, E, F). Half of children with generalized anxiety disorder will have another comorbid anxiety disorder.
   c. **Treatment**
      (1) A careful formulation, including an assessment of family dynamics, to develop an appropriate treatment plan

       (2) Treatment tends to be **psychotherapeutic** including possible family therapy, individual therapy, or use of relaxation techniques.

6. Obsessive–compulsive disorder (OCD)

  a. Overview. The criteria for OCD in children are the same as that in adults (see Chapter 21 II A) except that it is not required that children recognize the excessive nature of their fears. Onset is typically around 10 years of age. Boys and girls are equally affected. Symptoms tend to wax and wane with OCD, often persisting into adulthood.

  b. Differential diagnosis

    (1) Phobias, tic disorders, other anxiety disorders, substance use disorders, eating disorders, and psychotic disorders are included in the differential diagnosis. **Comorbid tic disorders are frequently seen.**

    (2) A subgroup of prepubertal children with OCD who present with an abrupt onset of symptoms following group B hemolytic streptococcal pharyngitis may have a syndrome known as **"PANDAS"** (Pediatric Autoimmune Neuropsychiatric Disorder Associated with Streptococcus). This is a recently described disorder in which antibodies to Streptococcus attack the basal ganglia. Investigational immunomodular and antibiotic treatments are being used.

  c. Treatment

    (1) Behavioral treatment, including exposure and response prevention, can be useful for adolescents and children who are motivated and cognitively able to participate.

    (2) Medications. SSRIs including fluoxetine (Prozac) and the tricyclic antidepressant clomipramine (Anafranil) may be useful.

7. Posttraumatic stress disorder (PTSD)

  a. Overview

    (1) PTSD is seen fairly frequently in the pediatric population. Index traumas may include exposure to natural disasters or war, or chronic exposure to abuse or domestic violence. DSM-IV criteria are the same as for adults except that children may reexperience the trauma through repetitive play, reenact the trauma through behavior, or have nightmares without recognizable content (see Chapter 20).

    (2) Symptoms may be acute or chronic. Early in the course of the disorder, children are likely to have difficulties with sleep and attention. Subsequently, trauma-specific and mundane fears may ensue, although with less of a tendency toward avoidance than adults with PTSD. Later still, children are likely to experience a foreshortened sense of the future. Children are less likely than adults to have flashbacks, but they may experience visual hallucinations or illusions, regression, irritability, hypervigilance, and an increased startle response.

HOT **KEY**

Asking the child about the scariest event in his or her life may help to elicit history relevant to a PTSD diagnosis.

---

b. Differential diagnosis. It is important to confirm that the index event(s) actually occurred. Adjustment disorder, acute stress disorder, OCD, substance use disorders, and psychotic disorders should also be considered.

c. Treatment

(1) Therapy may be individual, group, or family. Treatment includes allowing the child to ventilate feelings, especially soon after the trauma, psychoeducation, interpretation of defenses, creating perspective by creating a context for the trauma, desensitization, and finding ways to help the child regain a sense of control. The clinician should be alert to "anniversary reactions" to the traumatic event. Any ongoing exposure to trauma should be carefully assessed.

(2) Medications include the α-agonists guanfacine (Tenex), clonidine (Catapres), the β-blocker propranolol (Inderal), tricyclic antidepressants (TCAs), and SSRIs. The combination of clonidine and methylphenidate (Ritalin) has been associated with reports of sudden death.

II TIC DISORDERS. Tic disorders present before 18 years of age. To be considered a disorder, the symptoms must be associated with impairment. Tics caused by drugs or medical conditions must be ruled out.

A. Tourette's disorder

1. Overview. Tourette's disorder is characterized by multiple motor tics and at least one vocal tic (not necessarily concurrently), with symptoms lasting more than one year. Mean onset is at 7 years of age. Symptoms tend to peak at about 11 years of age and to improve by adulthood. The male-to-female ratio for Tourette's may be as high as 3:1. Generally, tics progress from simple motor (e.g., blinking or shrugging) to complex motor (including those tics that appear purposeful, e.g., brushing one's leg) to vocal. Rostral-to-caudal progression may occur.

HOT KEY

Tic symptoms tend to fluctuate with exacerbations in response to stress.

---

2. **Genetics.** This disorder tends to be autosomal dominant with a high degree of penetrance and variable expressivity.
3. **Neurophysiology.** Basal ganglia and corticothalamic pathways are involved, with dopaminergic pathways implicated.
4. **Differential diagnosis** includes Sydenham's chorea, Huntington's disease, Wilson's disease, postviral encephalitis, dyskinesias, substance use disorders, stereotypies (the repetition of senseless acts), and compulsive rituals. Tourette's and other tic disorders may also be associated with PANDAS (C 6 b (2)).
5. **Comorbidities are significant.** Approximately 50% of patients with Tourette's have comorbid ADHD; 30% have OCD (by early adolescence); 30% have conduct disorder; 30% have anxiety disorders; 30% have comorbid self-injurious behaviors.
6. **Treatment**
   a. **Educating** the child and family about the disorder and offering **support** can be very helpful. Support groups may be useful in addressing any ensuing social isolation.
   b. **Medication** should not be used unless symptoms are severe. If used, however, the choice of medication should be informed by comorbidities. Antipsychotics including haloperidol (Haldol), pimozide (Orap), and risperidone (Risperdal) are often used. Electrocardiograms must be followed for patients taking pimozide, with particular caution exercised at doses above 10 mg. Side effects should be strongly considered before starting children on antipsychotics. Clonidine and guanfacine are also used. Stimulants often exacerbate tics.
B. **Transient tic disorder.** This disorder lasts from weeks to months, but less than 12 months total, and generally involves simple motor tics. The male:female ratio is 3:1. This disorder may affect 5%–24% of school-aged children.
C. **Chronic motor or vocal tic disorder.** This disorder is less debilitating than Tourette's disorder. Unlike Tourette's, the patient has **either** vocal or motor tics, but not both. This disorder is rare

but occurs in the same families as Tourette's, and treatment is similar.

References

American Academy of Child and Adolescent Psychiatry: Practice parameters for the assessment and treatment of children and adolescents with anxiety disorders. *J Am Acad Child Adolesc Psychiatry* 36(695)(suppl 1): 69S–84S, 1997.

American Academy of Child and Adolescent Psychiatry: Practice parameters for the assessment and treatment of children and adolescents with posttraumatic stress disorder. *J Am Acad Child Adolesc Psychiatry* 37(9):997–1001, 1998.

Graske MG: Fear and anxiety in children and adolescents. *Bull Meninger Clin* 61(2) (suppl A): 1997.

King RA, Scahill L: The assessment and coordination of treatment of children and adolescents with OCD. *Child Adolesc Psychiatr Clin N Am* 8 (3):577–597, 1999.

41. Mood and Psychotic Disorders in Childhood and Adolescence

....

I **MOOD DISORDERS.** Mood disorders in childhood include **major depressive disorder, dysthymia,** and **bipolar disorder.** Children with depressive disorders are at greatly increased risk for anxiety disorders as well as substance use disorders, suicide, and disruptive behavior disorders. Girls and boys tend to be equally affected with mood disorders until adolescence, when girls are diagnosed more frequently.

A. Major depressive disorder
1. Clinical manifestations
  a. **DSM-IV criteria are the same for children as adults** (see Chapter 15 II B), except that mood may **be irritable rather than depressed** in children, and, rather than losing weight, children may simply **not make expected weight gains.**
  b. Pre- and postpubertal children often have different clinical manifestations (Table 41-1).
  c. Compared with adults with major depressive disorder, hallucinations are more frequent, while delusions are less frequent. Signs of melancholic depression (see Chapter 15 III A) are seen less frequently in children than in adults.

TABLE 41-1. Clinical Manifestations of Major Depressive Disorder in Prepubertal Versus Postpubertal Children

Prepubertal Children	Postpubertal Children
Tend to present with:	*Tend to present with:*
Psychomotor agitation	Hopelessness
Hallucinations	Anhedonia
Aggression	Delusions
Irritability	Hypersomnia
Moodiness	Psychomotor retardation
Somatic complaints	Changes in weight
Anxiety disorders (including separation anxiety disorder and phobias)	

Tom is an 8-year-old boy with a strong family history of depression who began to experience problems at school and at home associated with his parents' severe marital discord. Tom had frequent temper tantrums, fought with other children at school, and was described as "hyper." Tom had begun to eat very little, and frequently complained of stomachaches. On physical examination, he was sad and tearful and disclosed that he often thought about death, and at times heard "Chucky" tell him to do "bad things."

    d. Prevalence of major depression is 2% for children and 6% for adolescents.

2. Differential diagnosis
    a. Adjustment disorder with depressed mood
    b. Oppositional defiant disorder (see Chapter 42)
    c. Dysthymia
    d. Bipolar disorders
    e. Seasonal affective disorder
    f. Abuse and neglect
    g. Conduct disorder (see Chapter 42)
    h. Substance use disorders

3. Comorbidities
    a. Anxiety disorders (including separation anxiety disorder and phobias)

HOT KEY

Anxiety disorders in children are strongly associated with depressive disorders and may present with depressed mood.

    b. Substance use disorders
    c. Personality disorder symptoms may be present during the depressive episode but tend to remit with the depression.
    d. Conduct disorder symptoms may begin during the depressive episode but persist beyond it.
    e. Parental depression

4. Approach to the patient
    a. The physician should first **evaluate suicide potential.**
    b. Possible psychotic symptoms and **signs of bipolarity** must be assessed.
    c. Comorbid disorders should be explored, especially anxiety and substance use disorders.
    d. Family dynamics should be assessed, including possible depression in the patient's parents (a common co-

morbidity, especially in younger depressed patients), chaotic family environment, and other stressors.

- **e.** The child's **functioning in school** should be evaluated.
- **f.** **Indications for hospitalization** or partial hospitalization should be assessed.

5. Treatment is multifaceted.

- **a. Therapy**
  - **(1)** Cognitive behavioral therapy and interpersonal psychotherapy can be useful with adolescents.
  - **(2)** Family therapy and work with the child's school may be indicated.
- **b.** It is important to **treat comorbid conditions** and address psychosocial stressors.
- **c. Medication** may be indicated, particularly for severe, psychotic, and bipolar depression.
  - **(1)** Selective serotonin-reuptake inhibitors (SSRIs) are frequently used (see Chapter 16).
  - **(2)** Tricyclic antidepressants are often used but require baseline electrocardiograms (EKGs), with follow-up EKGs at levels above 3 mg/kg [1 mg/kg nortriptyline (NTP)] and liver function tests.
- **d. Maintenance treatment** is needed because major depressive disorder frequently recurs.

B. Dysthymic disorder

The diagnostic criteria for dysthymic disorder in children is the same as that used for adults except that the duration of symptoms need only be 1 year (see Chapter 15 III A). About 1% of children and approximately 4% of adolescents may have dysthymia. Symptoms tend to last about 4 years. Seventy percent of adolescents with dysthymia will eventually develop major depressive disorder, usually within 2–3 years. The approach to the patient and treatment for dysthymic disorder is similar to that for major depressive disorder.

C. Bipolar disorder, type I

1. Clinical manifestations. DSM-IV criteria for bipolar disorder are the same for children as adults (see Chapter 17 III A).

- **a.** Manic symptoms in younger school-aged children include irritability, impulsivity, distractibility, hyperactivity, prolonged tantrums, pressured speech, aggressivity, and lability.
- **b.** Older school-aged children and adolescents with mania may be disruptive, moody, explosive, euphoric, grandiose, paranoid, impulsive, and distractible, and may have pressured speech, flight of ideas, and insomnia.
- **c.** Up to 25% of children with major depression may go on to develop bipolar disorder within 5 years, especially if depression is severe or appears with psychotic features, psy-

chomotor retardation, acute onset, is associated with a strong family history of affective disorder, or if the manic decompensation is precipitated by medication.

    d. Bipolar disorder in children often includes delusions and hallucinations.

    e. About one-third of adults with bipolar disorder report symptoms in childhood.

2. Differential diagnosis

    a. Attention-deficit hyperactivity disorder (ADHD) (see Chapter 42). The extent to which the ADHD syndrome overlaps with mania is highly controversial.

    b. Conduct disorder (see Chapter 42)

    c. Substance use disorders

    d. Severe anxiety disorders

    e. Major depression with psychotic features or with psychomotor agitation

    f. Other psychotic disorders

    g. Impulse control disorders such as intermittent explosive disorder

    h. Schizophrenia (bipolar disorder is often misdiagnosed as schizophrenia in children, as it may present with marked psychotic symptoms)

3. Treatment is multifaceted.

    a. Medications

        (1) Lithium and **valproate** (Tegretol) tend to be first-line medications; **carbamazepine** (Depakote) is also used.

        (2) Valproate and carbamazepine are useful for mixed manic or rapid-cycling presentations. Valproate has been associated with polycystic ovarian syndrome, and therefore should be used with caution in girls.

        (3) Antipsychotics tend not to be useful for manic symptoms in children and adolescents.

    b. Supportive and psychoeducational work should be undertaken with the child and family.

    c. Educational interventions and social skills training are often needed.

    d. Individual psychotherapy may be needed to address problems that have arisen as a result of the disorder.

II PSYCHOTIC DISORDERS

A. Introduction

    1. The **nature of the psychotic symptoms is influenced by the child's developmental level.** The content of the delusions and hallucinations becomes more complex with increasing developmental stage.

        a. For example, the hallucinations or delusions of preschool or school-aged children may center around cartoon characters or identity issues.

b. In children under 10 years of age, delusions may be focused upon concerns of identity.

c. In older children, delusions may be somatic, religious, grandiose, persecutory, or involve ideas of reference.

d. Delusions during childhood are less systematized than in adulthood.

2. The **meaning of symptoms also depends upon the child's developmental stage.** Illogical thinking, looseness of associations, or magical thinking may be normal in preschool children, but may be abnormal when they occur in children over 6 or 7 years of age.

   a. **Preschool children may experience hallucinations while under stress,** particularly visual and tactile hallucinations at night, which **are not necessarily indicative of psychiatric disturbance.**

   b. In school age children, hallucinations tend to be less transient and more suggestive of psychopathology.

B. Schizophrenia

   1. Clinical manifestations

   a. **Criteria.** DSM-IV criteria for schizophrenia are essentially the same as that for adults (see Chapter 10 III A, B, C).

   b. **Premorbid signs** of schizophrenia may be seen **in 75% of pediatric cases,** including language difficulties, motor and neurological developmental difficulties, and odd personality styles.

   c. **Acute onset. In 25% of cases,** the disorder may present acutely in previously normal children.

   d. **Schizophrenia in children is rare.** Childhood schizophrenia tends to fit into one of two patterns.

   (1) **Very early onset schizophrenia (VEOS)** may be diagnosed if presentation is before 12 years of age. VEOS affects boys more often than girls, tends to present insidiously, and tends to include more prominent hallucinations, delusions, avolition (apathy), and poverty of speech.

   (2) **Early onset schizophrenia (EOS)** is diagnosed if presentation is between 12–18 years of age. EOS may be insidious or acute.

   (3) VEOS is seen much less frequently than EOS.

   e. **Peak onset of schizophrenia is late adolescence or early adulthood.**

   f. **Early onset** and **negative symptoms** may predict a **worse prognosis.**

   g. **Other signs and symptoms**

      (1) Auditory hallucinations occur in 80% of children with schizophrenia.

      (2) Visual and somatic hallucinations are also seen.

      (3) Delusions are experienced by 50% of children with schizophrenia.

      (4) Blunting of affect is common.

      (5) Thought disorder tends to be less prominent in children than in adults.

2. Differential diagnosis
—Bipolar disorder
—Major depressive disorder with psychotic features
—Schizophreniform disorder
—Schizoaffective disorder
—Conduct disorder
—Pervasive developmental disorder (PDD) spectrum disorders
—Language disorders
—Obsessive–compulsive disorder (OCD)
—Dissociative disorders
—Delirium
—Seizure disorder
—Central nervous system (CNS) pathology
—Neurodegenerative disorders (e.g., Huntington's chorea)
—Metabolic disorders (e.g., Wilson's disease)
—Endocrinopathies
—Toxic encephalopathies (e.g., substance abuse, medications including stimulants, heavy metals)

3. Approach to the patient
a. The physician should first assess the patient's level of safety.

b. A careful history, including birth and developmental history, premorbid social and academic functioning, family history, medical history, and history of affective and psychotic symptoms should be taken.

c. A full mental status exam should be performed.

d. A careful physical and neurologic evaluation should be done including electroencephalography (EEG).

e. Psychological testing should be considered, including assessments of intelligence, speech and language, academic achievement, projective testing, and adaptive functioning.

f. A toxicology screen should be performed on most children.

g. The presence of comorbid conditions should be assessed including learning and developmental disorders.

4. Treatment is multifaceted.
a. Antipsychotic medications including clozapine are used.

Children may be at increased risk of extrapyramidal symptoms (EPS) and neuroleptic malignant syndrome (NMS).

   b. Supportive and psychoeducational work should be undertaken with the child and family.

   c. Educational interventions and social skills training are generally needed.

C. Other psychotic disorders in childhood and adolescence include **major depression with psychotic features** (see I A) and **bipolar disorder with psychotic features** (see I C).

References

American Academy of Child and Adolescent Psychiatry: Practice parameters for the assessment and treatment of children and adolescents with depressive disorders. *J Am Acad Child Adolesc Psychiatry* 37(suppl 10):63S–83S, 1998.

McClellan J, Werry J: Practice parameters for the assessment and treatment of children and adolescents with schizophrenia. American Academy of Child and Adolescent Psychiatry. *J Am Acad Child Adolesc Psychiatry* 36 (suppl 10):177S–193S, 1997.

Schulz SC, Findling RL, Wise A, et al: Child and adolescent schizophrenia. *Psychiatr Clin N Am* 21(1):43–56, 1998.

42. Attention-Deficit/ Hyperactivity Disorder and Disruptive Behavior Disorders

> **HOT**
> ▶
> **KEY**
>
> Attention-deficit/hyperactivity disorder (ADHD), oppositional defiant disorder (ODD), and conduct disorder (CD) are a set of **interrelated, overlapping disorders.** All of these disorders **occur more frequently in boys** and **often in conjunction with problems with learning, speech and language,** and **aggression.**

I ATTENTION-DEFICIT/HYPERACTIVITY DISORDER (ADHD)

A. **Introduction.** ADHD has been diagnosed with increasing frequency in the United States. Current prevalence rates are about 4% in school-age children. It is diagnosed five times more frequently in boys than in girls.

B. **Defining characteristics**
1. ADHD is characterized by **symptoms of inattention and/or hyperactivity and impulsivity.**
2. It may be designated as **predominantly inattentive type, predominantly hyperactive–impulsive type,** or **combined type.**
3. Symptoms must be present earlier than 7 years of age (although the patient may not present for clinical attention until later), be present for at least 6 months, and impair functioning in at least two settings. For example, symptoms generally impair functioning in school, socially, at home, or all three.

C. **Clinical manifestations**
1. Children with **hyperactive–impulsive symptoms are generally identified earlier** than children with predominantly inattentive symptoms. Although symptomatic much earlier, children typically come to medical attention during the school-age years as symptoms become more apparent with the increased demands of a structured classroom.
2. It is important to **assess functioning in a variety of settings** rather than rely on clinical observations in the office setting to make the diagnosis, as highly structured activities, enjoy-

able activities, or frequent rewards can limit the expression of symptoms.

3. Course
   a. Symptoms may evolve from one type to another.
   b. One-third of cases remit during adolescence while two-thirds remit by adulthood.
   c. Up to 25% of adults with ADHD may develop antisocial personality disorder and 15% may develop substance use disorders, particularly patients still symptomatic by adulthood.
   d. Associated traumatic injuries are not uncommon (e.g., head injuries associated with the child's impulsivity).

D. Comorbidities
   1. Common comorbidities of ADHD
      a. ODD or CD (30%–50%)
      b. Depressive or anxiety disorders (15%–25%)
      c. Bipolar disorder (up to 20%)
      d. Tic disorders including Tourette's disorder (5%)
      e. Learning disorders (20%)
   2. It is unclear whether common risk factors account for the comorbidity, or whether difficulties resulting from the symptoms of ADHD symptoms contribute to development of some of the other disorders.
   3. Children with ADHD score lower on intelligence quotient (IQ) tests and may be at increased risk for learning and communication disorders.

E. Differential diagnosis
   1. Lead toxicity, absence seizures, fragile X syndrome, and postconcussion syndromes are medical disorders that may be associated with ADHD symptoms.
   2. Anxiety, mood, and disruptive behavior disorders are included in the differential diagnosis of ADHD.
   3. One should also consider that the patient may be exhibiting one of the following:
      a. Developmentally normal behaviors that may be distressing to caregivers
      b. Difficult behaviors that may be a normal response to an overstimulating or understimulating environment
      c. Symptoms related to the use of medications or illicit drugs
      d. Symptoms related to mental retardation

HOT KEY

Anxiety, in particular, may present with symptoms similar to ADHD in children.

F. Approach to the patient
 1. A **careful history** is essential and should focus on
    a. Birth and developmental history
    b. Neurologic review of systems
    c. Academic functioning
    d. Functioning in various settings
    e. Course of symptoms
    f. Stressors
    g. Associated symptoms
    h. Factors leading the family to seek clinical attention

HOT KEY Because ADHD is well known in the popular culture, families may already have labeled their child as having ADHD by the time they seek medical attention, and thus may be seeking a pill to cure what may be a more complex set of problems.

PROFILE Joel, a 7-year-old boy, has been having behavioral disturbances as a result of a depressive disorder triggered by a family stressor, namely his parents' divorce. Joel's symptoms have in turn added to the family's stress. The resultant family chaos and the boy's worsening self-esteem have exacerbated his behavioral symptoms. The parents have failed to properly identify this cycle and expect that a single ADHD medication will solve what is really a far more complex set of problems. Joel may or may not have ADHD, but a full assessment of the family situation is necessary to place his condition in proper context.

---

 2. A **psychiatric review of systems** (i.e., screening for symptoms of other disorders) and a careful **assessment of family functioning** are critical.
 3. **Clinical instruments and other evaluations**
    a. A scale often used to assess symptoms is the **Conners' Hyperactivity Rating Scale,** completed by both the parent and teacher. It can be helpful in both initial assessment and in assessing response to treatment. The **Child Behavior Checklist** may be helpful in assessing a range of difficulties.
    b. Cognitive, academic, or neuropsychological testing may be indicated to rule out comorbid learning disorders.
    c. A speech and language evaluation may be indicated to rule out a receptive language disorder. A hearing test may be indicated as well.

G. Treatment
 1. Nonpharmacological treatment is multifaceted.

    a. Psychoeducation should be included, with **family or individual psychotherapy** implemented as needed. Parents frequently need guidance regarding how to manage their child's difficult behaviors.

    b. Modifications in the child's educational program may need to be made.

    c. Behavioral interventions are important.

2. Comorbid psychiatric disorders should be addressed, including:

    a. Family functioning issues

    b. Issues that arise as a result of ADHD, such as poor self-esteem or other behavioral difficulties

3. Medications

    a. Stimulants. About 75% of children with ADHD improve with stimulants.

        (1) These include methylphenidate (Ritalin) (usually 0.3–0.7 mg/kg/dose given in morning and mid-day), sustained-release methylphenidate (Ritalin-SR) (same dosage range, given in morning), dextroamphetamine (Dexedrine) (usually 0.15–0.5 mg/kg given in morning and mid-day), sustained-release dextroamphetamine (Dexedrine Spansule), Adderall (usually 2.5–40 mg in morning and mid-day), and pemoline (Cylert) (dosage range 37.5–112.5 mg given in morning).

        (2) Pemoline has been associated with liver failure in 3% of patients.

        (3) Relative contraindications for stimulant use include psychosis, seizure disorder, tics, pervasive developmental disorder (PDD) spectrum disorders, cardiovascular conditions, other medications that may lead to drug–drug interactions, or substance abuse in the child or family member.

HOT **KEY**   Potential side effects of stimulants include loss of appetite, headache, psychotic symptoms, insomnia, irritability, dysphoria, abdominal pain, rebound symptoms, impaired cognition, growth impairment, tics, tachycardia, and hypertension.

---

    b. Nonstimulants

        (1) Tricyclic antidepressants, bupropion (Wellbutrin), and α-agonists clonidine (Catapres), and guanfacine (Tenex) are also used. Baseline and follow-up electrocardiograms (EKGs) and orthostatic blood pressures should be followed with α-agonists.

        (2) Nonstimulants should be selected on the basis of associated conditions (e.g., if the child also suffers from depressive symptoms, consider an antidepressant; if the child also has anxiety symptoms, consider an α-agonist).

II OPPOSITIONAL DEFIANT DISORDER (ODD) AND CONDUCT DISORDER (CD)

A. **Introduction.** These disorders **typically present in early adolescence.** Overall, they are **more commonly seen in boys:** 10% of boys and 5% of girls may be affected.

B. **Clinical manifestations**
1. **Oppositional defiant disorder** is characterized by a pattern of **negativistic, defiant, disobedient,** and **hostile behaviors.** Diagnostic criteria include 6 months of four symptoms associated with clinical impairment. The symptoms include losing one's temper, arguing with adults, defying adult rules, deliberately annoying others, blaming others, being easily annoyed by others, being resentful, and being vindictive.
2. **Conduct disorder** is characterized by a **pattern of violating the basic rights of others and/or violating major societal norms.** Behaviors associated with conduct disorder are more serious than those associated with oppositional defiant disorder.
   a. **Diagnostic criteria for CD** are divided into categories: aggression toward people or animals; destruction of property; deceitfulness or theft; or serious violations of rules.
   b. **Patients with CD generally have difficulty experiencing feelings of empathy, guilt, or remorse.**
      (1) Boys with these disorders tend to engage in more confrontational and aggressive behaviors than girls.
      (2) Specific behaviors are related to the child's developmental stage.
   c. **Course.** Up to 50% of children with CD may develop antisocial personality disorder as adults. They are at increased risk for substance abuse and personality, mood, anxiety, and somatoform disorders as adults.
   d. **Types.** Conduct disorder is of **childhood onset** if it presents before 10 years of age, and **adolescent onset** if it presents after 10 years of age.
      (1) Those with childhood-onset type tend to be more aggressive, male, have comorbid ADHD, and have previously met criteria for ODD. They often have a family history of antisocial personality disorder and substance abuse, and they are at increased risk of developing substance use disorders themselves.
      (2) Adolescent-onset type affects an increasing proportion of females, is often associated with an underlying

mood disorder for which patients self-medicate with drugs, and tends to have a better prognosis.

C. Causes. Psychosocial adversity factors are strongly correlated with ODD and CD. **Genetic, neuropsychiatric,** and **temperamental** factors also play a role.

D. Differential diagnosis and comorbidities of ODD and CD

HOT KEY

As children and adolescents have a limited repertoire by which to express distress, disruptive behaviors may be the final common pathway for a wide range of disturbances. Hence the differential diagnosis needs to be carefully considered for treatable conditions.

---

1. **Behaviors that are developmentally normal** at certain ages (e.g., oppositional behaviors during the pre-kindergarten and adolescent years) should be considered in the differential diagnosis.
2. **Mood disorders** including mania and depression, **psychotic disorders,** and **adjustment disorders** with disturbance of conduct should be ruled out.
3. Additionally, receptive language difficulties, mental retardation, and ADHD should be considered in the differential diagnosis of ODD.
4. **Comorbid conditions** are common (found in 70% of patients with CD) and include ADHD, posttraumatic stress disorder (PTSD), learning, language, mood and substance use disorders, and neurologic conditions.

E. Approach to the patient
1. The diagnoses of CD and ODD are primarily made by taking the history. As children will typically underreport symptoms, parents, teachers, probation officers, and guidance counselors may need to be contacted to get a complete history.
2. Screening for comorbid disorders is critical. Abuse and neglect should be carefully assessed, as should suicidal and homicidal ideation, particularly during periods of crisis.
3. The appropriateness of the child's educational program should also be evaluated.

F. Treatment
1. Multimodal treatment is usually optimal for ODD and CD. Unfortunately, the same psychosocial adversity factors that predispose patients to these disorders make treatment difficult.
2. Patients with these disorders may be involved with the juvenile justice system, with treatment carried out in this context. Treatment may also occur in the community, in a therapeu-

tic school, in a partial hospital or hospital setting, or in a residential facility.

3. Parent management training, behaviorally based programs, family therapy, and cognitive-behavioral interventions are frequently used with variable success.

4. It is important to actively treat comorbid and underlying disorders. Medications targeting aggressivity are used if other interventions are not effective, including antipsychotics (especially if the patient has paranoid ideation), mood stabilizers (especially if the patient has mood lability), and propranolol.

References

Cantwell DP: Attention deficit disorder: A review of the past 10 years. *J Am Acad Child Adolesc Psychiatry* 35(8):978–987, 1996.

Dulcan MK: Practice parameters for the assessment and treatment of children, adolescents and adults with attention deficit–hyperactivity disorder. *J Am Acad Child Adolesc Psychiatry* 36(suppl 10):85S–121S, 1997.

Steiner H: Practice parameters for the assessment and treatment of children and adolescents with conduct disorder. *J Am Acad Child Adolesc Psychiatry* 36(suppl 10):122S–139S, 1997.

43. Reactive Attachment Disorder

I **INTRODUCTION.** Reactive attachment disorder is a relatively uncommon but severe disorder that may be seen in children in the inpatient or outpatient setting.

II **CLINICAL MANIFESTATIONS**

A. Reactive attachment disorder consists of a syndrome of **pervasively impaired social relatedness.**
   1. It begins **before 5 years of age.**
   2. It is associated with **severely pathogenic early care** (i.e., lack of basic emotional or physical care, or lack of stable attachments).
B. **Types.** The disorder may be specified as either of two types.
   1. **Inhibited type** is characterized by inhibited, hypervigilant, or ambivalent social responsiveness.
   2. **Disinhibited type** children may be indiscriminately affectionate with strangers while being hostile or even aggressive with those to whom they feel closest.

III **CAUSES.** Reactive attachment disorder begins with a disturbance in the parent-child relationship, which leads to generalized social disability. **Risk factors** for the development of this disorder include institutionalization, parental inexperience, poverty, and neglect.

HOT KEY Not all children exposed to maltreatment will develop reactive attachment disorder. The child's temperament and constitution probably also play a role in the pathogenesis.

IV **DIFFERENTIAL DIAGNOSIS**

A. The **differential diagnosis** includes
   1. Pervasive developmental disorder (PDD) spectrum disorders
   2. Depressive disorders
   3. Posttraumatic stress disorder (PTSD) (if marked hypervigilant symptoms are present)

  4. Mental retardation
  5. Sensory deficits (such as blindness or deafness)
  6. Attention-deficit hyperactivity disorder (ADHD) (in the differential diagnosis for disinhibited type)
B. Comorbid conditions may include language and other developmental delays, feeding and eating disorders, failure to thrive (in infancy) and other growth disturbances, depressive disorders, and dissociative symptoms during periods of acute stress. Parental psychopathology and family dysfunction are often seen. Disruptive and aggressive behaviors and attentional difficulties may be associated, especially with disinhibited type. The behavioral difficulties may be associated with decreased frustration tolerance, impaired affect regulation, and disorganized thought processes.

V APPROACH TO THE PATIENT

A. To meet criteria for reactive attachment disorder, the child must be found to have social dysfunction that is pervasive as assessed by history, through collateral contacts, and on examination.
B. The psychiatric history should include asking about associated symptoms (see IV B), assessing for ongoing abuse and neglect, and noting presence of suicidal or assaultive potential.
C. A pediatric evaluation should be obtained, especially to note any concerns about eating or growth.
D. A complete social history should be taken that includes documentation of abuse and neglect. However, this may be difficult to obtain.
E. Cognitive testing, a speech and language evaluation, or both may be indicated.

VI TREATMENT

HOT KEY Placement in a stimulating, nurturing, and responsive setting is critical in treating symptoms associated with this disorder. However, the core symptoms of social dysfunction may be difficult to reverse.

A. Support and education about the disorder are usually indicated for family or caretakers.
B. Individual **psychotherapy** will often focus on interpersonal relationships. Psychotherapeutic work with the family or the dyad (the child and caretaker) may be indicated as well.
C. Medication may be used for associated psychiatric symptoms.
D. Educational support may be needed to address social and be-

havioral difficulties or any associated language or development delays.

References

Boris NW, Zeanah CH: Clinical disturbances of attachment in infancy and early childhood. *Curr Opin Pediatrics* 10(4):365–368, 1998.

Boris NW, Zeanah CH, Larrieu JA, et al: Attachment disorders in infancy and early childhood: A preliminary investigation of diagnostic criteria. *Am J Psychiatry* 155(2):295–297, 1998.

44. Elimination Disorders

I ELIMINATION DISORDERS

A. Although most elimination disorders have psychological components, it is important to rule out medical pathology in the course of evaluating the child.

B. In the absence of a specific medical etiology, consider the disorder a symptom of individual psychological or family conflict. Encopresis, in the absence of organic pathology, can be seen as a psychological solution to an emotional conflict.

C. Elimination disorders are often comorbid with other childhood psychiatric disorders.

D. A child psychiatrist may be involved in treating these disorders, often in consultation with a pediatrician.

II ENURESIS

A. **Introduction**

1. Enuresis is defined as **failure of bladder control** beyond the age when a child should be developmentally capable of continence.

2. **Types**

a. Enuresis can be **nocturnal** (nighttime) or **diurnal** (daytime). Since nocturnal enuresis is much more common, it is the focus of this section.

b. Enuresis may also be **primary** or **secondary.**

(1) **Primary enuresis** is when the child has never achieved continence.

(2) **Secondary enuresis** occurs when the child has had at least 3 months of continence before having episodes of incontinence.

3. Attainment of urinary continence is a developmental milestone. Failure to achieve this milestone can leave children feeling embarrassed and humiliated.

 HOT KEY Attainment of urinary continence is part of a developmental spectrum. Therefore, there is a great deal of variability in the age at which a child is able to remain dry.

---

4. **Epidemiology.** The prevalence of nocturnal enuresis is estimated to be 7% of 8-year-olds with a 1% decrease with each

year of age. Boys with this disorder slightly outnumber girls. If one parent had enuresis, a child has a 40% likelihood of having the disorder, and if both parents had enuresis, a child has a 70% likelihood of having it. Ninety percent of children achieve daytime continence by 4 years of age, and 90% achieve nighttime continence by 8 years of age.

B. Causes. In most cases, an exact cause of enuresis cannot be determined.

1. The most common causes of enuresis include:
   a. Genetic causes: This is a disorder that runs in families
   b. Maturational delay
   c. Small bladder capacity
   d. Sleep patterns: Parents often report that their children are very heavy sleepers and "don't wake up in time."
   e. Faulty training: Children who are physically and emotionally ready can attain bladder continence. A child who is pushed too hard or parents who are too punitive in their approach to toilet training often cause control battles that parents cannot win.
   f. Emotional factors: Children with emotional difficulties may develop enuresis.
   g. Urinary tract infections
   h. Decreased bladder size secondary to constipation
   i. Consumption of liquids containing caffeine, which has a diuretic effect
   j. Sickle cell disease
2. Less common causes of enuresis include:
   a. Diabetes mellitus and diabetes insipidus
   b. Spinal cord abnormalities, including tethered spinal cord
   c. Ectopic ureters

C. Approach to the patient

1. A **thorough history** includes assessment of the following:
   a. The reason that the family is seeking help at the current time
   b. Each parent's and the child's understanding of the problem
   c. The child's degree of motivation to remain dry
   d. Previous efforts to address the enuresis
   e. The usefulness of these efforts and their effects on the child's self-esteem
   f. The pattern of the enuretic symptoms (e.g., weekdays versus weekends)
   g. Family history of enuresis (understanding the family history can help to put the problem in perspective for the child)
2. A thorough **physical, neurologic,** and **genital examination** should be performed on a child with enuresis.

3. **Laboratory investigation** should be limited to a urinalysis and urine culture (especially for girls). The history and physical examination should guide other laboratory tests ordered.
D. **Treatment.** There are many approaches to the treatment of enuresis. Spontaneous cure rates are reported in up to 15% of cases per year, but this does not mean families should just wait it out. Children are embarrassed and humiliated by this problem and deserve a treatment approach. Treatment will not be successful without the full involvement and participation of the child, including taking responsibility for the problem and involvement in attempting to solve it. Punitive techniques are not useful or effective and will only prolong the problem.
   1. **Supportive measures**
      a. Education demystifies the problem for children and helps establish motivation.
      b. Education also eases family conflict.
      c. Reassurance is helpful; children are often relieved to know that this is a common problem and that it will not last forever.
      d. All children eventually achieve urinary continence. Families should be educated that there are no immediate, quick fixes, and that they should expect relapses.
   2. **Practical measures**
      a. The child should take developmentally appropriate steps to clean up in the morning, such as pulling off wet sheets or changing their own pajamas.
      b. If the child awakens in the middle of the night, they might place a towel on their bed.
      c. Diapers and disposable training pants should be avoided after 4 years of age because they inhibit motivation.
      d. The patient should reduce fluid intake at and after dinner and empty the bladder before bed.
      e. Attempts should be made to cure diurnal enuresis first. This is usually the easier of the two forms to treat.
   3. **Behavioral measures**
      a. Bladder stretching with urgency containment exercises. This approach is best used for diurnal enuresis. It has been reported to have a 30%–35% cure rate.
      b. Motivational techniques involve establishing a reward system for each dry night. This can be established with star charts or calendar stickers. This approach stresses the importance of the child taking responsibility for solving the problem and uses positive feedback for success. It is best used as an adjunct to other therapies.
      c. Wetness alarms have a success rate of 70%–80% with a relapse rate of 10%. They must be used every night and

may awaken parents as well. Training is required to use the alarm properly.

  4. **Medications**
    a. Desmopressin acetate **(DDAVP)**, an antidiuretic, has an initial success rate of 50%, but a very high relapse rate of 90%. It is not a good choice for a first-line treatment, unless it is used for special situations such as sleepovers or camp.
    b. **Imipramine** is a tricyclic antidepressant with the same initial success rate and relapse rate as DDAVP. It has cardiac side effects when taken in high doses.
    c. Oxybutynin is an anticholinergic, antispasmodic bladder muscle relaxant. It is used mostly to treat diurnal enuresis.
  5. If after 4–8 months of dedicated treatment the child is still wetting, there may be underlying psychosocial stressors for which enuresis is a maladaptive solution, which should be explored.

III ENCOPRESIS

A. **Introduction**
  1. **Definition.** Encopresis is the **involuntary repeated passage of stool in inappropriate places.** It must occur at least once per month for 3 months after a child has reached 4 years of age. and such passage may not be directly related to a medical etiology. About 2% of children suffer from encopresis.

HOT KEY

Children and families often feel hopeless and ashamed about the problem and often try to keep it a secret.

  2. **Types**
    a. **Primary encopresis** occurs when the child fails to attain continence.
    b. **Secondary encopresis** is diagnosed when there has been a significant period of continuous continence prior to the development of incontinence.
B. **Clinical manifestations**
  1. The primary manifestation of encopresis is the soiling of underwear.
  2. Children may also complain of recurrent abdominal pain.
  3. Up to 25% of children with encopresis also have enuresis due to decreasing bladder capacity and residual urine volumes from pressure on the adjacent colon.
  4. Urinary tract infections are common in girls with encopresis.

C. Pathophysiology and cause
  1. **Stool retention** leads to chronic constipation and encopresis.
  2. Factors that may lead to stool retention include the following:
      a. Genetic tendency toward slow gut motility
      b. Temperament
      c. Autonomy struggles
      d. Toilet training issues (e.g., punitive measures)
      e. Psychosocial stress
      f. Medications that slow gut motility
      g. Busy schedules (with consequent infrequent toileting)
      h. Avoidance of school bathrooms
      i. Lack of patience (e.g., in children with ADHD, see Chapter 42).
      j. History of trauma, such as sexual abuse
  3. **Mechanism** of constipation and encopresis
      a. When stool is retained in the rectal vault, it becomes large, hard, and painful to pass. This leads to further retention. Liquid stool is able to pass around the solid stool mass, which leads to soiling of the child's underwear.
      b. As a consequence of the large amount of stool in the rectum, the bowel becomes stretched and there is decreased nerve sensation. Children are unaware that they should move their bowels and often become desensitized to their own odor.

D. Differential diagnosis. In children who have encopresis, it is important to rule out organic pathology.
  1. **Hirschsprung's disease** is a rare condition that can lead to stool retention.
  2. Other organic causes of stool retention include **hypothyroidism** or **impairment of voluntary muscle control,** which may occur with children who have cerebral palsy, spinal cord lesions, or spina bifida.
  3. Certain medications (e.g., narcotics, tricyclics, and diuretics such as caffeine) may also lead to chronic constipation.

E. Approach to the patient
  1. A **thorough history** of the problem should be taken.
      a. Any early potentiating factors should be included.
      b. Current and past attempts to manage the problem should be noted.
      c. The physician must investigate whether there are psychosocial stressors present for the child and family, including ruling out the possibility of sexual abuse.
  2. A complete **physical, neurologic,** and **rectal examination** is required to rule out organic pathology.
  3. **Abdominal films** can confirm stool retention.
  4. Manometric studies should be done if there is a suspicion of Hirschsprung's disease.
  5. Pediatric consultation may be indicated.

F. Treatment

    1. Education and demystification are the initial steps in treatment. It helps to reduce the tension often seen in families of children who have encopresis. Families should be made aware that:

        a. Children are ashamed of soiling and often hide their underwear.

        b. Children with encopresis lose the ability to sense rectal fullness, are unaware of fecal leakage, and are desensitized to their odor.

        c. Fecal soiling is not a deliberate act.

HOT KEY

The child and parents must all be motivated to solve the problem. Without the child's participation, the program will not be successful.

---

    2. Restoring proper bowel function

        a. The bowel must be allowed to return to its normal size and regain sensation. This may take many months.

        b. This restoration is initiated by cleaning out the bowel, which may be done on an outpatient basis unless there are concerns about compliance or obstructive symptoms. It can be done from "above" (i.e., oral medications) or from "below" (i.e., rectally), with pediatric consultation as needed.

    3. Maintenance

        a. Once bowel catharsis has been established, it is important to initiate a bowel continence maintenance program. The goals are:

            (1) No soiling

            (2) Regular bowel movements in the toilet

            (3) An improved ability to sense the urge to have a bowel movement

        b. To achieve and maintain these goals, a bowel continence program should consist of:

            (1) Stool softener

            (2) Daily multivitamin, if the child is treated with mineral oil for an extended period of time

            (3) Daily toilet sitting for at least 10 minutes twice a day, especially after meals

            (4) Increased activity and a high fiber diet

            (5) Motivational techniques such as star charts or calendar stickers

    4. Supportive measures

        a. Punitive techniques must be avoided. The child must feel empowered to achieve success.

b. Parents and doctors serve as coaches to help the process.
c. Underlying psychosocial issues must be addressed concurrently.
d. Setbacks are to be expected. This is a chronic problem with frequent relapses.

References

Loening-Baucke V: Encopresis and soiling. *Pediatr Clin North Am* 43(1):279–298, 1996.
Moffatt M: Nocturnal enuresis: A review of the efficacy of treatments and practical advice of clinicians. *J Dev Behav Pediatr* 18(1):49–56, 1997.
Schmitt BD: Nocturnal enuresis. *Pediatr Rev* 18(6):183–190, 1997.

PART XIV

GERIATRIC PSYCHIATRY

45. Normal Aging and Assessment of the Older Adult

I **INTRODUCTION.** Cognitive and physical changes occurring in healthy, active older people (over 55 years of age) may be minimal. However, the overall incidence of physical and mental impairments increases with age, as does the use of medications. Chapter 45 reviews the normal correlates of the aging process. These should be kept in mind in evaluating and treating any older patient.

HOT KEY Sensory impairments, medical illnesses, and the losses that accompany advancing age (e.g., death of a spouse, social isolation) increase the likelihood of psychiatric disturbances in the older adult.

II **CLINICAL CONSEQUENCES OF NORMAL AGING**

A. **Central nervous system changes**
 1. The ability to process and rapidly respond to novel information **declines.**
 2. Slight **deterioration occurs in stored memories** and in the ability to perform tasks that require a person's cumulative life experience and knowledge.
 3. **Sensory impairments occur,** chiefly hearing and vision loss. These are the most common underlying causes of problems in communication, and they predispose the patient to psychiatric disturbances (e.g., depression, paranoia, confusion).
 4. **Personality continues to develop** into the last years of life, shaped by the challenges of older age.
B. **Physiologic changes**
 1. **Decline in cardiovascular function** (diminished cardiac out-

put) occurs and leads to reduced blood flow to brain and other vital organs, **slowing pharmacokinetics.**

2. Age-related **adrenergic changes** reduce compensatory heart rate increases in the face of hypotension, **making drug-induced hypotension more likely.**

3. **Reduced responsiveness to hypoxia and hypercapnia** exacerbates the respiratory depressant effects of sedating medications.

4. **Gastrointestinals mucus secretion** is reduced, increasing the incidence of dry mouth and constipation.

5. **The liver's ability to metabolize medications is decreased,** and there is a decline in total body water and increase in body fat, causing **medications to be distributed differently.**

6. **Sleep lightens,** tends to be interrupted, and the circadian rhythm shifts to earlier bedtimes and waketimes.

HOT

Increased age predisposes a patient to much greater sensitivity to medications and the need for lower doses.
KEY

III APPROACH TO ASSESSING THE OLDER PATIENT. A **thorough evaluation** is essential in the geriatric patient, because of the higher incidence of comorbid medical and psychiatric illnesses in the elderly population, as well as cognitive impairment. Here are some guidelines for performing a careful assessment:

A. The patient should be **interviewed alone,** and the physician must take the time to hear what the patient has to say.

B. The physician must **be sensitive to hearing impairment** by making sure to speak slowly and clearly.

C. The patient's family and other **collateral sources should be interviewed,** to explore any history of psychiatric symptoms or cognitive decline.

D. A **complete medical history** should be taken, including all current and recently changed medications, special diets and supplements, and sleep aids.

E. The patient should be questioned about **present and past alcohol or substance use.** Alcohol use in the elderly is commonly overlooked, and alcohol abuse is easily missed. The patient's family should also be questioned about a possible history of alcohol abuse.

F. The physician should search for undiagnosed medical problems, drug interactions, occult injury (e.g., head injuries caused

HOT KEY

About 10% of men and 1% of women over 65 years of age have been alcohol dependent at some time in their lives.

by falls), or psychosocial stressors to account for unexplained symptoms.

G. Appropriate cognitive, mood, and functional assessment scales should be used to help correctly define the patient's impairments.

IV TREATMENT CONSIDERATIONS AND FOLLOW-UP

A. **Treatment for sensory impairment** is essential to preserve the patient's functional ability and quality of life.

B. Clearly, **preventive health care measures** are essential at this age.

C. **Addressing the psychosocial issues of late life**—social isolation, loss of income, death of spouse—may go a long way toward preserving the patient's mental health. The aging person may benefit from **"reminiscence therapy"**—a type of life review that helps the person to frame his life conceptually and confront mortality. This form of therapy capitalizes on the universal tendency of people to reminisce with friends and family, leading to conscious evaluation and resolution of intrapsychic or interpersonal conflicts.

References

Fleming MF, LB Manwell, KL Barry, et al: Brief physician advice for alcohol problems in older adults: A randomized community-based trial. *J Fam Pract* 48(5):378–384, 1999.

Kirby M, Denihan A, Bruce I, et al: Benzodiazepine use among the elderly in the community. *Int J Geriatr Psychiatry* 14(4):280–284, 1999.

Zec RF: The neuropsychology of aging. *Exp Gerontol* 30(3–4):431–442, 1995.

46. Depression in Older Adults

I **INTRODUCTION.** The onset of mood disturbances in older adults (over 65 years of age) is common, though probably less prevalent than onset in younger adults. Still, major depression has a prevalence of 1%–4% in all persons over 65 years of age. The rates are much higher in the hospital setting. As many as 30% of hospitalized elderly patients have significant depressive symptoms. New-onset mania in the geriatric population is rare, but does occur, especially in people who have a previous history of depression.

II **CLINICAL MANIFESTATIONS OF MAJOR DEPRESSION IN OLDER ADULTS**

A. Depression in older adults presents clinically in much the same way as it does in younger adults (see Chapter 15), but some differences are apparent. **Older adults are more likely to:**
  1. Focus on somatic complaints
  2. Appear anxious
  3. Minimize the presence of depressed mood ("masked depression")
  4. Minimize feelings of guilt
  5. Suffer from psychotic symptoms
B. Morbid worrying and hypochondriacal concerns are frequently seen in patients in the geriatric setting without a clear DSM-IV diagnosis of depression; however, in patients with major depression, hypochondriasis represents a risk factor for suicide. **Elderly white men have a high rate of suicide** (45.6 per 100,000) compared with elderly African-American men (16.2 per 100,000), elderly white women (7.5 per 100,000), or elderly African-American women (2.4 per 100,000).
C. **The morbidity associated with depression is higher in the geriatric population.** For example, weight loss from loss of appetite can lead to the need for hospitalization and place the patient at increased risk for infection and other medical problems.

III **CAUSES OF MAJOR DEPRESSION IN OLDER ADULTS**

A. The **primary risk factors** for depression in the older adult are:
  1. A past history of depression
  2. Physical illness or chronic pain

3. Life stressors—such as the death of a spouse, friend, or other loved one
4. Social isolation
5. Medications (Table 46-1)

TABLE 46-1. Medications that May Trigger Depression	
Reserpine	Clonidine
Methyldopa	Hydralazine
Propranolol	Cimetidine
Digitalis	Corticosteroids
Indomethacin	Propoxyphene
Codeine	Antibiotics
Levodopa	Tamoxifen
Vincristine	Vinblastine
Benzodiazepines	Barbiturates

B. Certain medical illnesses are especially likely to prompt depressive or anxious symptoms.
   1. **Chronic obstructive pulmonary disease (COPD).** Panic, anxiety, and mood symptoms related to dyspnea, chronic hypoxemia, and hypercapnia may be comorbid with COPD. The β-agonists and corticosteroids used to treat the lung disease may also prompt depression.
   2. **Myocardial infarction and congestive heart failure.** The loss of physical vitality associated with these disorders predispose the patient to depressive symptoms, and untreated or undertreated major depression increases the patient's risk of premature death from heart disease symptoms.
   3. **Cancer.** Major depression sometimes develops in patients with paraneoplastic syndromes (inappropriate endocrine secretion from tumors) even before cancer is diagnosed. Pancreatic, oat cell carcinoma, and others are thought to be especially likely to do this. Patients with other cancers may also be predisposed to depression; the stress of facing a life-threatening illness increases the risk of depressive symptoms.
   4. **Parkinson's disease, stroke,** and other **neurological diseases** including **dementia** all predispose the patient to major depression.
   5. **Endocrinopathies,** especially **hypo- and hyperthyroidism** and Cushing's disease, can predispose patients to major depression.
C. **Psychosocial stressors** can be important contributors to depressive symptoms. Factors such as limited mobility, separation from family or friends, poor financial resources, or difficult living conditions all confer a risk toward the development of major depression.

HOT

KEY

The presence of social support is a strong predictor of recovery from depression.

IV DIFFERENTIAL DIAGNOSIS

A. The tendency of elderly patients with depression to **minimize or even deny depressed mood** may complicate the task of assessing the patient. In older patients with depression, the symptoms of social withdrawal, loss of interest in activities, and a preoccupation with somatic complaints are more likely to be verbalized.

B. Patients also may exhibit cognitive impairment; some even appear to be demented. This "pseudodementia" is the result of cognitive slowing caused by depression and is fully reversible with antidepressant treatment. It is important to consider underlying medical or comorbid psychiatric illnesses that may also be present.

V APPROACH TO THE PATIENT

A. The evaluation guidelines in Chapter 45 will help you begin your assessment of the older patient.

B. The possible presence of cognitive impairment requires the use of Folstein's **Mini-Mental State Examination** (see Table 3-1) in any older adult with psychiatric illness, but especially someone with depression.

C. It may also be helpful to administer the **Geriatric Depression Scale** (see Table 46-2) to quantify depressive symptoms.

VI SOMATIC TREATMENT.   Many modalities of treatment may be useful in the treatment of geriatric depression. Most often, medications are necessary, but don't overlook the importance of other therapies.

A. Antidepressant medications

   1. Selective serotonin reuptake inhibitors are better tolerated than most other classes of antidepressants. Sertraline (Zoloft) (50–100 mg every day) is a good choice. Fluoxetine should be used with caution because of its long half-life. Paroxetine (Paxil) and fluvoxamine maleate (Luvox) have potential for drug-drug interactions due to cytochrome P450 or protein-binding effects.

   2. Tricyclic antidepressants—nortriptyline (50–75 mg every day) is the most useful agent in this class, as it has limited anticholinergic side effects.

TABLE 46-2. Geriatric Depression Scale (Short Version)

Answers indicating depression are boldfaced. Each answer counts for 1 point; scores greater than 5 indicate probable depression.

1.	Are you basically satisfied with your life?	YES/**NO**
2.	Have you dropped many of your activities and interests?	**YES**/NO
3.	Do you feel that your life is empty?	**YES**/NO
4.	Do you often get bored?	**YES**/NO
5.	Are you in good spirits most of the time?	YES/**NO**
6.	Are you afraid that something bad is going to happen to you?	**YES**/NO
7.	Do you feel happy most of the time?	YES/**NO**
8.	Do you often feel helpless?	**YES**/NO
9.	Do you prefer to stay at home, rather than going out and doing new things?	**YES**/NO
10.	Do you feel you have more problems with memory than most?	**YES**/NO
11.	Do you think it is wonderful to be alive now?	YES/**NO**
12.	Do you feel pretty worthless the way you are now?	**YES**/NO
13.	Do you feel full of energy?	YES/**NO**
14.	Do you feel that your situation is hopeless?	**YES**/NO
15.	Do you think that most people are better off than you are?	**YES**/NO

Special Instructions: The scale can be used as a self-rating or observer-rated instrument. It has also been used as an observer-rated scale in mildly demented subjects.

From Yesavage JA: Geriatric depression scale. *Psychopharmacol Bull* 24:709, 1988. Used with permission.

3. Other antidepressants

   a. Venlafaxine (75 mg every day to 75 mg three times a day) may be administered; monitor for elevations in blood pressure.

   b. Nefazadone—Because of its potential for sedation and confusion, "start low and go slow" (50 mg every day, or 50 mg twice a day, increased to 100–300 mg a day in divided doses over a month).

4. Monoamine oxidase (MAO) inhibitors—These have high potential for causing falls due to hypotension, and for drug-drug interactions, but are highly efficacious. Phenelzine sulfate (Nardil) (45 mg daily) or tranylcypromine sulfate (Parnate) (30–40 mg daily) should be considered.

5. Stimulants—In low doses (e.g., 5 mg methylphenidate every morning and noon) these are often helpful in reversing apathy and improving appetite. They also have the additional advantage of working within days (rather than weeks) after treatment is initiated.

HOT KEY

Because the onset of antidepressant effect is usually later in elderly patients, an adequate trial of medication requires 6–9 weeks of treatment.

B. Antipsychotic medications may be required if significant paranoia, delusions, or other psychotic disturbances are manifest. Avoid low-potency medications (e.g., chlorpromazine) due to the potential for hypotension. Low doses of high-potency medications (e.g., haloperidol, risperidone) are the treatments of choice.

C. Electroconvulsive therapy (ECT) is an effective treatment, especially for psychotic or agitated depression (see Chapter 15 II H 4). It is also safe in elderly patients who have not had recent cardiac illness or intracranial lesions. Follow-up may include maintenance ECT to prevent relapse.

 NONSOMATIC TREATMENT Cognitive-behavioral and interpersonal psychotherapy have been found to be effective in mild cases of depression. Group therapy can offer benefits to depressed, isolated patients. Addressing psychosocial stressors, especially grief and other symptoms of loss, is especially important. Incorporating the family into treatment is essential, as the family is often the source of emotional support and frequently provides day-to-day support in functioning as well.

References

Flint AJ, Rifat SL: Recurrence of first-episode geriatric depression after discontinuation of maintenance antidepressants. *Am J Psychiatry* 156(6):943–945, 1999.

Lebowitz BD, Pearson JL, Schneider LS, et al: Diagnosis and treatment of depression in late life. Consensus statement update. *JAMA* 278(14):1186–1190, 1997.

Yaffe K, Blackwell T, Gore R, et al: Depressive symptoms and cognitive decline in nondemented elderly women: A prospective study. *Arch Gen Psychiatry* 56(5):425–430, 1999.

47. Dementia

I **INTRODUCTION.** Older adults commonly experience forgetfulness and may be concerned about the implications. Problems with recall are normal for advanced age, and such age-related impairment does not progress to dementia. An older person's brain can be very sensitive, and the onset of illness, the effects of medications, or even a change in the environment (e.g, hospitalization) can prompt severe cognitive disturbances. These disturbances must be differentiated from dementia. It is important to perform a thorough evaluation of the patient and collect collateral information to clearly determine the patient's diagnosis and his or her functional capacity.

HOT
▶
KEY

Dementia tends to be chronic, slowly progressive, and largely irreversible and is due to one of a few categories of disease. Delirium tends to be acute, largely reversible if diagnosed promptly, and can be due to one of several different categories of disease.

II **CLINICAL MANIFESTATIONS OF DEMENTIA**

A. **Diagnostic criteria**
   1. **Memory impairment**
   2. **Deficits in at least one other cognitive domain**
   3. **Significant social** or **occupational dysfunction** as a result of the impairment or deficit
B. **Behavior changes that frequently accompany dementia**
   1. Agitation (anxious, angry, or confused behavior), frequently occuring in the evening or at night ("sundowning")
   2. Paranoia
   3. Insomnia (problem maintaining sleep) is common.
C. The time course of these changes is gradual—**over months or years** rather than hours or days (as is characteristic of delirium).
D. **Progression**
   1. **Mild** dementia symptoms may cause mostly subjective impairment in short-term memory and language (forgetting names, problems with word-finding, the need to make lists).
   2. As the dementia progresses to **moderate** levels, the decline in cognition may cause the patient to get lost in a familiar

neighborhood or place himself in harm's way by doing such things as forgetting to turn off the stove.

3. **Severe** dementia manifests as near total loss of memory, including remote memory, necessitating constant supervision and assistance with all aspects of self-care.

III CAUSES OF DEMENTIA

A. **Alzheimer's disease** is the **most common cause** of dementia, and it affects 5%–10% of people over 65 years of age. Genetic risk factors are possible, and some cases appear familial; all cases affect cholinergic transmission. Dementia of the Alzheimer's type is of insidious onset and shows early symptoms of memory loss, leading to progressive deterioration in judgment and abstract thinking, language, and visual-spatial skills. There is eventual impairment in gait, extrapyramidal symptoms, incontinence, and, ultimately, death.

B. **Vascular dementia** is the second most common cause of dementia. It is characterized by a stepwise (rather than insidious) decline in cognitive function as small infarctions take place. Focal neurological signs or symptoms are usually present, and patients have a history of hypertension. Neuroimaging studies usually help make the diagnosis.

C. **Parkinson's disease** frequently leads to cognitive deterioration that usually follows clear motor symptoms. Patients may have more prominent difficulty in initiating tasks or problem solving than that seen in patients with Alzheimer's disease. Comorbid depressive symptoms are also common.

D. **Huntington's disease** occurs in 4–7 per 100,000 people. It is of autosomal dominant inheritance. Cell death in the neostriatum prompts the onset of choreiform movement, dementia, and psychiatric disturbances, especially depression.

E. **Pick's disease** (also called Niemann-Pick's disease) is a rare presenile dementia with predominant frontal lobe impairment. Progressive decline in memory and cognitive function occurs over 2–10 years. Transmission is probably genetic.

F. **Creutzfeldt-Jakob disease.** An infectious agent (prion) causes a rapidly progressive cognitive decline, leading to death within months of the onset of symptoms.

IV DIFFERENTIAL DIAGNOSIS

A. **Differentiating acute from chronic cognitive impairment** is the first step in evaluating any new patient with suspected dementia.

1. **Delirium** is an **acute, reversible** cause of cognitive change and is common in the hospital setting. Delirium is **often misdiag-**

nosed as dementia, especially if no family members are present to attest to the patient's usually normal mental status. Evaluation of patients with known long-term memory impairment is more commonly performed in the outpatient setting.

2. The following are the most common causes of delirium:

   a. Metabolic: vitamin deficiencies, hyponatremia, hypercalcemia, hypo- or hyperglycemia, low oxygen or elevated carbon dioxide, uremic or hepatic encephalopathy

   b. Vascular: stroke, subdural, or epidural hematoma

   c. Endocrine: hyper- or hypothyroidism, hyperparathyroidism, Cushing's disease, or Addison's disease

   d. Seizure: postictal confusion is very common

   e. Trauma: concussion, postconcussive syndrome

   f. Uremic or hepatic encephalopathy

   g. Infectious causes: infections anywhere in the body, but especially meningitis, encephalitis, pneumonia, or urinary tract infection

   h. Medications: including anticholinergic medications, antihypertensives, corticosteroids, digitalis, phenytoin (Dilantin), nonsteroidal anti-inflammatory agents (NSAIDs), sedative hypnotics

B. Rule out underlying psychiatric disorders

1. Dementia syndrome of **depression**—also called "pseudodementia"—is characterized by psychomotor retardation, apathy, and cognitive impairment. Frequently, the complaint of memory loss is worse than the actual memory impairment (i.e., if the depression is cured, the memory will come back).

2. **Anxiety** can present as confusion and cognitive impairment, and can especially interfere with memory and concentration.

3. **Psychotic disorders**—disorganization, paranoia, or delusions—may impair concentration, reality testing, and functional status.

4. **Alcohol dependence**—intoxication or withdrawal states may present with delirium that resolves slowly, mimicking a dementing disorder. Patients with alcohol dependence may also present with symptoms of thiamine deficiency called Wernicke's syndrome (nystagmus, ataxia, and memory problems). If untreated, this syndrome can lead to irreversible memory impairment.

C. The **metabolic disorders** that may prompt delirium are important to consider first, since some may be life-threatening (e.g, hypo- or hypernatremia, hypoglycemia, or hypercalcemia).

D. An **infection** can present with confusion. An infection as seemingly minimal as cystitis can present with confusion (and often incontinence) rather than complaints such as pain on urination.

E. Sensory impairment or **hospitalization** can cause sufficient confusion to mimic a dementing disorder.

V APPROACH TO THE PATIENT

A. The guidelines in Chapter 45 (III) should be followed in beginning your evaluation of the older adult patient with possible dementia.

B. There are no clinical tests to prove Alzheimer's disease is present (except postmortem brain examinations). A diagnosis of dementia of the Alzheimer's type cannot be made until other potential causes of dementia have been ruled out based on the patient's **history, physical examination,** and **comorbid symptoms.**

C. It is essential to be patient, speak clearly, and use a translator if not speaking the patient's primary language. While maintaining sensitivity, it is also essential not to shy away from asking the right questions. Asking these questions is vital to obtaining a correct diagnosis.

D. The Mini-Mental State Examination (see Table 3-1) is easy to perform at the bedside. A full neurological assessment is necessary to investigate a vascular etiology.

VI TREATMENT. Once other causes of cognitive change have been eliminated, the **choice of treatment depends on the underlying cause** of dementia.

A. Vascular dementia requires preventive treatment with anti-clotting medications [e.g., aspirin 325–650 mg orally each day, or warfarin sodium (Coumadin)] if appropriate to prevent further infarctions.

B. Alzheimer's disease deficits may be minimized for a time by treatment with anticholinesterase inhibitors [tacrine or donepezil (Aricept) (5–10 mg orally once daily)], though the eventual downhill course is inevitable.

C. Dementia associated with Parkinson's disease may be slowed by treatments for other Parkinson's symptoms.

D. In all cases, **supportive and preventive** health care are backbones to your treatment.

E. Low-dose, high-potency neuroleptics [e.g,. risperidone (Risperdal) 0.5–2.0 mg] are the treatment of choice for the agitation, insomnia, and paranoia that are frequent consequences of dementia. These are the drugs of choice because of the lack of anticholinergic effects, including hypotension, and minimal interactions with other medications.

VII FOLLOW-UP AND REFERRAL

A. **Neuropsychological testing** may help delineate the patient's functional capacities.

B. A **long-term care plan is ultimately essential** in the life of a demented individual.

    1. The **early identification of a health care proxy, durable
power of attorney,** and **creation of a living will** are all important aspects of the patient's care.

    2. Many patients' families care for them in their home, though
this can be a significant burden with time. **The most difficult
aspect of patient care by the family tends to be the disrupted
sleep patterns common in moderate to severely dementing
illnesses.** It is this factor, more often than any other, that often prompts removal of the patient to an extended care facility.

References

Geerlings MI, Jonker C, Bouter LM, et al: Association between memory complaints
and incident Alzheimer's disease in elderly people with normal baseline cognition.
Am J Psychiatry 156(4):531–537, 1999.

Patterson C, et al.: The recognition, assessment, and management of dementing disorders: Conclusions from the Canadian Consensus Conference on Dementia. CMAJ
160(suppl 12):S1–15, 1999.

Pryse-Phillips W: Do we have drugs for dementia? No. *Arch Neurol* 56(6):735–737,
1999.

APPENDIX:
DSM-IV Classification

....

NOS = Not Otherwise Specified.

An *x* appearing in a diagnostic code indicates that a specific code number is required.

An ellipsis (...) is used in the names of certain disorders to indicate that the name of a specific mental disorder or general medical condition should be inserted when recording the name (e.g., 293.0 Delirium Due to Hypothyroidism).

If criteria are currently met, one of the following severity specifiers may be noted after the diagnosis:

> Mild
> Moderate
> Severe

If criteria are no longer met, one of the following specifiers may be noted:

> In Partial Remission
> In Full Remission
> Prior History

DISORDERS USUALLY FIRST DIAGNOSED IN INFANCY, CHILDHOOD, OR ADOLESCENCE

MENTAL RETARDATION

Note: These are coded on Axis II. (see Multiaxial System at end of this appendix)

317	Mild Mental Retardation
318.0	Moderate Mental Retardation
318.1	Severe Mental Retardation
318.2	Profound Mental Retardation
319	Mental Retardation, Severity Unspecified

LEARNING DISORDERS

315.00	Reading Disorder
315.1	Mathematics Disorder
315.2	Disorder of Written Expression
315.9	Learning Disorder NOS

MOTOR SKILLS DISORDER

315.4	Developmental Coordination Disorder

COMMUNICATION DISORDERS

315.31	Expressive Language Disorder
315.31	Mixed Receptive Expressive Language Disorder
315.39	Phonological Disorder
307.0	Stuttering
307.9	Communication Disorder NOS

PERVASIVE DEVELOPMENTAL DISORDERS

299.0	Autistic Disorder
299.80	Rett's Disorder
299.10	Childhood Disintegrative Disorder
299.80	Asperger's Disorder
299.80	Pervasive Developmental Disorder NOS

ATTENTION-DEFICIT AND DISRUPTIVE BEHAVIOR DISORDERS

314.xx	Attention-Deficit/Hyperactivity Disorder
.01	Combined Type
.00	Predominantly Inattentive Type
.01	Predominantly Hyperactive-Impulsive Type
314.9	Attention-Deficit/Hyperactivity Disorder NOS

312.8 Conduct Disorder
Specify type: Childhood-Onset
Type/Adolescent-Onset
Type
313.81 Oppositional Defiant
Disorder
312.9 Disruptive Behavior Disorder
NOS

FEEDING AND EATING DISORDERS OF INFANCY OR EARLY CHILDHOOD

307.52 Pica
307.53 Rumination Disorder
307.59 Feeding Disorder of Infancy or
Early Childhood

TIC DISORDERS

307.23 Tourette's Disorder
307.22 Chronic Motor or Vocal Tic
Disorder
307.21 Transient Tic Disorder
Specify if: Single Episode/Recurrent
307.20 Tic Disorder NOS

ELIMINATION DISORDERS

—.— Encopresis
787.6 With Constipation and Overflow Incontinence
307.7 Without Constipation and
Overflow Incontinence
307.6 Enuresis (Not Due to a General Medical Condition)
Specify type: Nocturnal
Only/Diurnal Only/Nocturnal
and Diurnal

OTHER DISORDERS OF INFANCY, CHILDHOOD, OR ADOLESCENCE

309.21 Separation Anxiety Disorder
Specify if: Early Onset
313.23 Selective Mutism
313.89 Reactive Attachment Disorder
of Infancy or Early Childhood
Specify type: Inhibited
Type/Disinhibited Type
307.3 Stereotypic Movement Disorder
Specify if: With Self-Injurious
Behavior
313.9 Disorder of Infancy, Childhood, or Adolescence NOS

DELIRIUM, DEMENTIA, AND AMNESTIC AND OTHER COGNITIVE DISORDERS

DELIRIUIM

293.0 Delirium due to . . . [*Indicate
the General Medical Condition*]
—.— Substance Intoxication Delirium
(*refer to Substance-Related Disorders for substance-specific
codes*)
—.— Substance Withdrawal Delirium
(*refer to Substance-Related Disorders for substance-specific
codes*)
—.— Delirium Due to Multiple Etiologies (*code each of the specific etiologies*)
780.09 Delirium NOS

DEMENTIA

290.xx Dementia of the Alzheimer's
Type, With Early Onset
(*also code 331.0 Alzheimer's
Disease on Axis III*)
.10 Uncomplicated
.11 With Delirium
.12 With Delusions
.13 With Depressed Mood
Specify if: With Behavioral Disturbance

290.xx Dementia of the Alzheimer's
Type, With Late Onset
(*also code 331.0 Alzheimer's
disease on Axis III*)
.0 Uncomplicated
.3 With Delirium
.20 With Delusions
.21 With Depressed Mood
Specify if: With Behavioral disturbance
290.xx Vascular Dementia
.40 Uncomplicated
.41 With Delirium
.42 With Delusions
.43 With Depressed Mood
Specify if: With Behavioral disturbance
294.9 Dementia Due to HIV Disease
(*also code 043.1 HIV infection
affecting central nervous system
on Axis III*)
294.1 Dementia Due to Head
Trauma
(*also code 854.00 head injury
on Axis III*)
294.1 Dementia Due to Parkinson's
Disease (*also code 332.0
Parkinson's disease on Axis III*)

294.1   Dementia Due to Huntington's Disease (*also code 333.4 Huntington's disease on Axis III*)

290.10 Dementia Due to Pick's *Disease* (*also code 331.1 Pick's disease on Axis III*)

290.10 Dementia Due to Creutzfeldt-Jakob Disease (*also code 046.1 Creutzfeldt-Jakob disease on Axis III*)

294.1   Dementia Due to . . . [*Indicate the General Medical Condition not listed above*] (*also code the general medical condition on Axis III*)

—.—   Substance-Induced Persisting Dementia (*refer to Substance-Related Disorders for substance-specific codes*)

—.—   Dementia Due to Multiple Etiologies (*code each of the specific etiologies*)

294.8   Dementia NOS

AMNESTIC DISORDERS

294.0   Amnestic Disorder Due to. . . [*Indicate the General Medical Condition*] Specify if: Transient/Chronic

—.—   Substance-Induced Persisting Amnestic Disorder (*refer to Substance-Related Disorders for substance-specific codes*)

294.8   Amnestic Disorder NOS

OTHER COGNITIVE DISORDERS

294.9   Cognitive Disorder NOS

MENTAL DISORDERS DUE TO A GENERAL MEDICAL CONDITION NOT ELSEWHERE CLASSIFIED

293.89 Catatonic Disorder Due to . . . [*Indicate the General Medical Condition*]

310.1   Personality Change Due to . . . [*Indicate the General Medical Condition*] *Specify type:* Labile Type/Disinhibited Type/Aggressive Type/Apathetic Type/Paranoid Type/Other Type/Combined Type/Unspecified type

293.9   Mental Disorder NOS Due to . . . [*Indicate the General Medical Condition*]

SUBSTANCE-RELATED DISORDERS

[a]The following specifiers may be applied to Substance Dependence:

> With Physiological Dependence/Without Physiological Dependence
> Early Full Remission/Early Partial Remission
> Sustained Full Remission/Sustained Partial Remission
> On Agonist Therapy/In a Controlled Environment

The following specifiers apply to Substance-Induced Disorders as noted:

> [I]With Onset During Intoxication/[W]With Onset During Withdrawal

ALCOHOL-RELATED DISORDERS

Alcohol Use Disorders

303.90 Alcohol Dependence[a]
305.00 Alcohol Abuse

Alcohol-Induced Disorders

303.00 Alcohol Intoxication
291.8   Alcohol Withdrawal
            Specify if: With Perceptual Disturbances
291.0   Alcohol Intoxication Delirium

291.0   Alcohol Withdrawal Delirium
291.2   Alcohol-Induced Persisting Dementia
291.1   Alcohol-Induced Persisting Amnestic Disorder
291.x   Alcohol-Induced Psychotic Disorder
   .5   With Delusions[I,W]
   .3   With Hallucinations[I,W]
291.8   Alcohol-Induced Mood Disorder[I,W]
291.8   Alcohol-Induced Anxiety Disorder[I,W]

291.8   Alcohol-Induced Sexual Dys-
            function[I]
291.8   Alcohol-Induced Sleep
            Disorder[I,W]
291.9   Alcohol-Related Disorder
            NOS

AMPHETAMINE (OR AMPHETA-MINE-LIKE)-RELATED DISORDERS

Amphetamine Use Disorders

304.40 Amphetamine Dependence[a]
305.70 Amphetamine Abuse

Amphetamine-Induced Disorders

292.89 Amphetamine Intoxication
            Specify if: With Perceptual
            Disturbances
292.0   Amphetamine Withdrawal
292.81 Amphetamine Intoxication
            Delirium
292.xx Amphetamine-Induced Psy-
            chotic Disorder
    .11 With Delusions[I]
    .12 With Hallucinations[I]
292.84 Amphetamine-Induced Mood
            Disorder[I,W]
292.89 Amphetamine-Induced Anxi-
            ety Disorder[I]
292.89 Amphetamine-Induced Sexual
            Dysfunction[I]
292.89 Amphetamine-Induced Sleep
            Disorder[I,W]
292.9   Amphetamine-Related Disor-
            der NOS

CAFFEINE-RELATED DISORDERS

Caffeine-Induced Disorders

305.90 Caffeine Intoxication
292.89 Caffeine-Induced Anxiety
            Disorder[I]
292.89 Caffeine-Induced Sleep
            Disorder[I]
292.9   Caffeine-Related Disorder NOS

CANNABIS-RELATED DISORDERS

Cannabis Use Disorders

304.30 Cannabis Dependence[a]
305.20 Cannabis Abuse

Cannabis-Induced Disorders

292.89 Cannabis Intoxication
            Specify if: With Perceptual Dis-
            turbances
292.81 Cannabis Intoxication Delirium

292.xx Cannabis-Induced Psychotic
            Disorder
    .11 With Delusions[I]
    .12 With Hallucinations[I]
292.89 Cannabis-Induced Anxiety Dis-
            order[I]
292.9   Cannabis-Related Disorder NOS

COCAINE-RELATED DISORDERS

Cocaine Use Disorders

304.20 Cocaine Dependence[a]
305.60 Cocaine Abuse

Cocaine-Induced Disorders

292.89 Cocaine Intoxication
            Specify if: With Perceptual Dis-
            turbances
292.0   Cocaine Withdrawal
292.81 Cocaine Intoxication Delirium
292.xx Cocaine-Induced Psychotic
            Disorder
    .11 With Delusions[I]
    .12 With Hallucinations[I]
292.84 Cocaine-Induced Mood Disor-
            der[I,W]
292.89 Cocaine-Induced Anxiety Dis-
            order[I,W]
292.89 Cocaine-Induced Sexual Dys-
            function[I]
292.89 Cocaine-Induced Sleep Disor-
            der[I,W]
292.9   Cocaine-Related Disorder
            NOS

HALLUCINOGEN-RELATED DISORDERS

Hallucinogen Use Disorders

304.50 Hallucinogen Dependence[a]
305.30 Hallucinogen Abuse

Hallucinogen-Induced Disorders

292.89 Hallucinogen Intoxication
292.89 Hallucinogen Persisting Per-
            ception Disorder (Flashbacks)
292.81 Hallucinogen Intoxication
            Delirium
292.xx Hallucinogen-Induced Psy-
            chotic Disorder
    .11 With Delusions[I]
    .12 With Hallucinations[I]
292.84 Hallucinogen-Induced Mood
            Disorder[I]
292.89 Hallucinogen-Induced Anxiety
            Disorder[I]
292.9   Hallucinogen-Related Disorder
            NOS

INHALANT-RELATED DISORDERS

Inhalant Use Disorders

304.60   Inhalant Dependence[a]
305.90   Inhalant Abuse

Inhalant-Induced Disorders

292.89   Inhalant Intoxication
292.81   Inhalant Intoxication Delirium
292.82   Inhalant-Induced Persisting Dementia
292.xx   Inhalant-Induced Psychotic Disorder
   .11   With Delusions[I]
   .12   With Hallucinations[I]
292.84   Inhalant-Induced Mood Disorder[I]
292.89   Inhalant-Induced Anxiety Disorder[I]
292.9   Inhalant-Related Disorder NOS

NICOTINE-RELATED DISORDERS

Nicotine Use Disorder

305.10   Nicotine Dependence[a]

Nicotine-Induced Disorder

292.0   Nicotine Withdrawal
292.9   Nicotine-Related Disorder NOS

OPIOID-RELATED DISORDERS

Opioid Use Disorders

304.00   Opioid Dependence[a]
305.50   Opioid Abuse

Opioid-Induced Disorders

292.89   Opioid Intoxication
       Specify if: With Perceptual Disturbances
292.0   Opioid Withdrawal
292.81   Opioid Intoxication Delirium
292.xx   Opioid-Induced Psychotic Disorder
   .11   With Delusions[I]
   .12   With Hallucinations[I]
292.84   Opioid-Induced Mood Disorder[I]
292.89   Opioid-Induced Sexual Dysfunction[I]
292.89   Opioid-Induced Sleep Disorder[I,W]
292.9   Opioid-Related Disorder NOS

PHENCYCLIDINE (OR PHENCYCLIDINE-LIKE)-RELATED DISORDERS

Phencyclidine Use Disorders

304.90   Phencyclidine Dependence[a]
305.90   Phencyclidine Abuse

Phencyclidine-Induced Disorders

292.89   Phencyclidine Intoxication
       Specify if: With Perceptual Disturbances
292.81   Phencyclidine Intoxication Delirium
292.xx   Phencyclidine-Induced Psychotic Disorder
   .11   With Delusions[I]
   .12   With Hallucinations[I]
292.84   Phencyclidine-Induced Mood Disorder[I]
292.89   Phencyclidine-Induced Anxiety Disorder[I]
292.9   Phencyclidine-Related Disorder NOS

SEDATIVE-, HYPNOTIC-, OR ANXIOLYTIC-RELATED DISORDERS

Sedative, Hypnotic, or Anxiolytic use Disorders

304.10   Sedative, Hypnotic, or Anxiolytic Dependence[a]
305.40   Sedative, Hypnotic, or Anxiolytic Abuse

Sedative-, Hypnotic-, or Anxiolytic-Induced Disorders

292.89   Sedative, Hypnotic, or Anxiolytic Intoxication
292.0   Sedative, Hypnotic, or Anxiolytic Withdrawal
       Specify if: With Perceptual Disturbances
292.81   Sedative, Hypnotic, or Anxiolytic Intoxication Delirium
292.81   Sedative, Hypnotic, or Anxiolytic Withdrawal Delirium
292.82   Sedative-, Hypnotic-, or Anxiolytic-Induced Persisting Dementia
292.83   Sedative-, Hypnotic-, or Anxiolytic-Induced Persisting Amnestic Disorder
292.xx   Sedative-, Hypnotic-, or Anxiolytic-Induced Psychotic Disorder
   .11   With Delusions[I,W]
   .12   With Hallucinations[I,W]
292.84   Sedative-, Hypnotic-, or Anxiolytic-Induced Mood Disorder[I,W]
292.89   Sedative-, Hypnotic-, or Anxiolytic-Induced Anxiety Disorder[W]
292.89   Sedative-, Hypnotic-, or

Anxiolytic-Induced Sexual
Dysfunction[I]

292.89   Sedative-, Hypnotic-, or
Anxiolytic-Induced Sleep
Disorder[I,W]

292.9   Sedative-, Hypnotic-, or Anxi-
olytic-Related Disorder NOS

POLYSUBSTANCE-RELATED DISORDER

304.80   Polysubstance Dependence[a]

OTHER (OR UNKNOWN) SUBSTANCE-RELATED DISORDERS

Other (or Unknown) Substance Use Disorders

304.90   Other (or Unknown) Substance Dependence[a]

305.90   Other (or Unknown) Substance Abuse

Other (or Unknown) Substance-Induced Disorders

292.89   Other (or Unknown) Substance Intoxication
Specify if: With Perceptual Disturbances

292.0   Other (or Unknown) Substance Withdrawal
Specify if: With Perceptual Disturbances

292.81   Other (or Unknown) Substance-Induced Delirium

292.82   Other (or Unknown)
Substance-Induced Persisting
Dementia

292.83   Other (or Unknown) Substance-Induced Persisting
Amnestic Disorder

292.xx   Other (or Unknown) Substance-
Induced Psychotic Disorder
   .11   With Delusions[I,W]
   .12   With Hallucinations[I,W]

292.84   Other (or Unknown) Substance-Induced Mood
Disorder[I,W]

292.89   Other (or Unknown) Substance-
Induced Anxiety Disorder[I,W]

292.89   Other (or Unknown) Substance-Induced Sexual Dysfunction[I]

292.89   Other (or Unknown) Substance-
Induced Sleep Disorder[I,W]

292.9   Other (or Unknown)
Substance-Related Disorder
NOS

SCHIZOPHRENIA AND OTHER PSYCHOTIC DISORDERS

295.xx   Schizophrenia

*The following Classification of Longitu-
dinal Course applies to all subtypes of
Schizophrenia.*

Episodic With Interepisode
Residual Symptoms (*Specify if:*
With Prominent Negative
Symptoms/Episodic With No
Interepisode Residual Symptoms)
Continuous (*Specify if:* With
Prominent Negative Symptoms.
Single Episode In Partial
Remission (*Specify if:* With
Prominent Negative Symptoms/
Single Episode In Full Remission)
Other or Unspecified Pattern

   .30   Paranoid Type
   .10   Disorganized Type
   .20   Catatonic Type
   .90   Undifferentiated Type
   .60   Residual Type

295.40   Schizophreniform Disorder
Specify if: Without Good Prog-

nostic Features/With Good
Prognostic Features

295.70   Schizoaffective Disorder
Specify type: Bipolar Type/De-
pressive Type

297.1   Delusional Disorder
Specify type: Erotomanic
Type/Grandiose Type/Jealous
Type/Persecutory Type/Somatic
Type/Mixed Type/Unspecified
Type

298.8   Brief Psychotic Disorder
Specify if: With Marked Stres-
sor(s)/Without Marked Stres-
sor(s)/With Postpartum
Onset

297.3   Shared Psychotic Disorder

293.xx   Psychotic Disorder Due
to . . .
[*Indicate the General Medical
Condition*]
   .81   With Delusions
   .82   With Hallucinations

——.—   Substance-Induced Psychotic
Disorder (*refer to Substance-*

*Related Disorders for sub-
stance-specific codes)*
Specify if: With Onset During
Intoxication/With Onset During Withdrawal
298.9 Psychotic Disorder NOS

MOOD DISORDERS

*Code current state of Major Depressive
Disorder or Bipolar I Disorder in fifth
digit:*
1 Mild
2 Moderate
3 Severe without Psychotic
Features
4 Severe With Psychotic Features
Specify: Mood-Congruent Psychotic Features/Mood-Incongruent
Psychotic Features
5 In Partial Remission
6 In Full Remission
0 Unspecified
*The following specifiers apply (for cur-
rent or most recent episode) to Mood Disorders as noted:*
[a]Severity/Psychotic/Remission
Specifiers/[b]Chronic/[c]With Catatonic
Features/[d]With Melancholic Features/
[e]With Atypical Features/[f]With Postpartum Onset
*The following specifiers apply to Mood
Disorders as noted:*
[g]With or Without Full Interepisode
Recovery/[h]With Seasonal Pattern/
[i]With Rapid Cycling

DEPRESSIVE DISORDERS

296.xx Major Depressive Disorder,
.2x Single Episode[a,b,c,d,e,f]
.3x Recurrent[a,b,c,d,e,f,g,h]
300.4 Dysthymic Disorder
Specify if: Early Onset/Late
Onset

Specify: With Atypical Features
311 Depressive Disorder NOS

BIPOLAR DISORDERS

296.xx Bipolar I Disorder
.0x Single Manic Episode[a,c,f]
Specify if: Mixed
.40 Most Recent Episode Hypomanic[g,h,i]
.4x Most Recent Episode
Manic[a,c,f,g,h,i]
.6x Most Recent Episode
Mixed[a,c,f,g,h,i]
.5x Most Recent Episode Depressed[a,b,c,d,e,f,g,h,i]
.7 Most Recent Episode Unspecified[g,h,i]
296.89 Bipolar II Disorder[a,b,c,d,e,f,g,h,i]
*Specify (current or most recent
episode):* Hypomanic/
Depressed
301.13 Cyclothymic Disorder
296.80 Bipolar Disorder NOS
293.83 Mood Disorder Due to . . .
[*Indicate the General Medical
Condition*]
Specify type: With Depressive
Features/With Major
Depressive-Like Episode/With
Manic Features/With Mixed
Features
—.— Substance-Induced Mood Dis-
order
(refer to Substance-Related
Disorders for substance-specific
codes)
Specify type: With Depressive
Features/With Manic
Features/With Mixed
Features
Specify if: With Onset During
Intoxication/With Onset
During Withdrawal
296.90 Mood Disorder NOS

ANXIETY DISORDERS

300.01 Panic Disorder Without Agoraphobia
300.21 Panic Disorder With Agoraphobia
300.22 Agoraphobia Without History
of Panic Disorder
300.29 Specific Phobia
Specify type: Animal Type/Nat-
ural Environment Type/Blood-
Injection-Injury Type/Situa-
tional Type/Other Type
300.23 Social Phobia
Specify if: Generalized
300.3 Obsessive-Compulsive Disorder
Specify if: With Poor Insight
309.81 Posttraumatic Stress Disorder
Specify if: Acute/Chronic
Specify if: With Delayed Onset

308.3   Acute Stress Disorder
300.02 Generalized Anxiety Disorder
293.89 Anxiety Disorder Due to . . .
            [*Indicate the General Medical Condition*]
            Specify if: With Generalized Anxiety/With Panic Attacks/With Obsessive-Compulsive Symptoms
—.—   Substance-Induced Anxiety Disorder (*refer to Substance-*

Related Disorders for substance-specific codes)
Specify if: With Generalized Anxiety/With Panic Attacks/With Obsessive-Compulsive Symptoms/With Phobic Symptoms
Specify if: With Onset During Intoxication/With Onset During Withdrawal
300.00 Anxiety Disorder NOS

SOMATOFORM DISORDERS

300.81 Somatization Disorder
300.81 Undifferentiated Somatoform Disorder
300.11 Conversion Disorder

Specify type: With Motor Symptom or Deficit/With Sensory Symptom or Deficit/With Seizures or Convulsions/With Mixed Presentation

307.xx Pain Disorder

.80   Associated With Psychological Factors
.89   Associated With Both Psychological Factors and a General Medical Condition
           Specify if: Acute/Chronic
300.7 Hypochondriasis
           Specify if: With Poor Insight
300.7 Body Dysmorphic Disorder
300.81 Somatoform Disorder NOS

FACTITIOUS DISORDERS

300.xx Factitious Disorder
   .16 With Predominantly Psychological Signs and Symptoms
   .19 With Predominantly Physical Signs and Symptoms

.19   With Combined Psychological and Physical Signs and Symptoms
300.19 Factitious Disorder NOS

DISSOCIATIVE DISORDERS

300.12 Dissociative Amnesia
300.13 Dissociative Fugue
300.14 Dissociative Identity Disorder

300.6 Depersonalization Disorder
300.15 Dissociative Disorder NOS

SEXUAL AND GENDER IDENTITY DISORDERS

SEXUAL DYSFUNCTIONS

The following specifiers apply to all primary Sexual Dysfunctions:

Lifelong Type/Acquired Type
Generalized Type/Situational Type
Due to Psychological Factors/Due to Combined Factors

Sexual Desire Disorders

302.71 Hypoactive Sexual Desire Disorder
032.79 Sexual Aversion Disorder

Sexual Arousal Disorders

302.72 Female Sexual Arousal Disorder
302.72 Male Erectile Disorder

Orgasmic Disorders

302.73 Female Orgasmic Disorder
302.74 Male Orgasmic Disorder
302.75 Premature Ejaculation

Sexual Pain Disorders

302.76 Dyspareunia (Not Due to a General Medical Condition)

306.51 Vaginismus (Not Due to a General Medical Condition)

Sexual Dysfunction Due to a General Medical Condition

625.8 Female Hypoactive Sexual Desire Disorder Due to . . . [*Indicate the General Medical Condition*]
608.89 Male Hypoactive Sexual Desire Disorder Due to . . . [*Indicate the General Medical Condition*]
607.84 Male Erectile Disorder Due to . . . [*Indicate the General Medical Condition*]
625.0 Female Dyspareunia Due to . . . [*Indicate the General Medical Condition*]
608.89 Male Dyspareunia Due to . . . [*Indicate the General Medical Condition*]
625.8 Other Female Sexual Dysfunction Due to . . . [*Indicate the General Medical Condition*)
608.89 Other Male Sexual Dysfunction Due to . . . [*Indicate the General Medical Condition*]
—.— Substance-Induced Sexual Dysfunction (*refer to Substance-Related Disorders for substance-specific codes*) *Specify if:* With Impaired Desire/With Impaired Arousal/With Impaired Orgasm/With Sexual Pain *Specify if:* With Onset During Intoxication
302.70 Sexual Dysfunction NOS

PARAPHILIAS

302.4 Exhibitionism
302.81 Fetishism
302.89 Frotteurism
302.2 Pedophilia *Specify if:* Sexually Attracted to Males/Sexually Attracted to Females/Sexually Attracted to Both *Specify if:* Limited to Incest *Specify type:* Exclusive Type/Nonexclusive Type
302.83 Sexual Masochism
302.84 Sexual Sadism
302.3 Transvestic Fetishism *Specify if:* With Gender Dysphoria
302.82 Voyeurism
302.9 Paraphilia NOS

GENDER IDENTITY DISORDERS

302.xx Gender Identity Disorder
.6 in Children
.85 in Adolescents or Adults *Specify if:* Sexually Attracted to Males/Sexually Attracted to Females/Sexually Attracted to Both/Sexually Attracted to Neither
302.6 Gender Identity Disorder NOS
302.9 Sexual Disorder NOS

EATING DISORDERS

307.1 Anorexia Nervosa *Specify type:* Restricting Type; Binge-Eating/Purging Type
307.51 Bulimia Nervosa *Specify type:* Purging Type/Nonpurging Type
307.50 Eating Disorder NOS

SLEEP DISORDERS

PRIMARY SLEEP DISORDERS
Dyssomnias

307.42 Primary Insomnia
307.44 Primary Hypersomnia *Specify if:* Recurrent
347 Narcolepsy
780.59 Breathing-Related Sleep Disorder
307.45 Circadian Rhythm Sleep Disorder *Specify type:* Delayed Sleep Phase Type/Jet Lag Type/Shift Work Type/Unspecified Type
307.47 Dyssomnia NOS

Parasomnias

307.47 Nightmare Disorder
307.46 Sleep Terror Disorder

307.46 Sleepwalking Disorder
307.47 Parasomnia NOS

SLEEP DISORDERS RELATED TO ANOTHER MENTAL DISORDER

307.42 Insomnia Related to . . .
          [*Indicate the Axis I or Axis II Disorder*]
307.44 Hypersomnia Related to . . .
          [*Indicate the Axis I or Axis II Disorder*]

OTHER SLEEP DISORDERS

780.xx Sleep Disorder Due to . . .
          [*Indicate the General Medical Condition*]

.52 Insomnia Type
.54 Hypersomnia Type
.59 Parasomnia Type
.59 Mixed Type
—.— Substance-Induced Sleep Disorder
          (*refer to Substance-Related Disorders for substance-specific codes*)
          Specify type: Insomnia Type/Hypersomnia Type/ Parasomnia Type/Mixed Type
          Specify if: With Onset During Intoxication/With Onset During Withdrawal

IMPULSE-CONTROL DISORDERS NOT ELSEWHERE CLASSIFIED

312.34 Intermittent Explosive Disorder
312.32 Kleptomania
312.33 Pyromania
312.31 Pathological Gambling
312.39 Trichotillomania
312.30 Impulse-Control Disorder NOS

ADJUSTMENT DISORDERS

309.xx Adjustment Disorder
   .0 With Depressed Mood
  .24 With Anxiety
  .28 With Mixed Anxiety and Depressed Mood
   .3 With Disturbance of Conduct
   .4 With Mixed Disturbance of Emotions and Conduct
   .9 Unspecified
          Specify if: Acute/Chronic

PERSONALITY DISORDERS

Note: These are coded on Axis II.
301.0 Paranoid Personality Disorder
301.20 Schizoid Personality Disorder
301.22 Schizotypal Personality Disorder
301.7 Antisocial Personality Disorder
301.83 Borderline Personality Disorder
301.50 Histrionic Personality Disorder
301.81 Narcissistic Personality Disorder
301.82 Avoidant Personality Disorder
301.6 Dependent Personality Disorder
301.4 Obsessive-Compulsive-Personality Disorder
301.9 Personality Disorder NOS

OTHER CONDITIONS THAT MAY BE A FOCUS OF CLINICAL ATTENTION

PSYCHOLOGICAL FACTORS AFFECTING MEDICAL CONDITON

316 . . . [*Specified Psychological Factor*] Affecting . . . [*Indicate the General Medical Condition*]
          Choose name based on nature of factors:

Mental Disorder Affecting Medical Condition
Psychological Symptoms Affecting Medical Condition
Personality Traits or Coping Style Affecting Medical Condition
Maladaptive Health Behaviors Affecting Medical Condition

Stress-Related Physiological Response Affecting Medical Condition

Other or Unspecified Psychological Factors Affecting Medical Condition

MEDICATION-INDUCED MOVEMENT DISORDERS

332.1	Neuroleptic-Induced Parkinsonism
333.92	Neuroleptic Malignant Syndrome
333.7	Neuroleptic-Induced Acute Dystonia
333.99	Neuroleptic-Induced Acute Akathisia
333.82	Neuroleptic-Induced Tardive Dyskinesia
333.1	Medication-Induced Postural Tremor
333.90	Medication-Induced Movement Disorder NOS

OTHER MEDICATION-INDUCED DISORDER

995.2	Adverse Effects of Medication NOS

RELATIONAL PROBLEMS

V61.9	Related Problem Related to a Mental Disorder or General Medical Condition
V61.20	Parent-Child Relational Problem
V61.1	Partner Relational Problem
V61.8	Sibling Relational Problem
V62.81	Relational Problem NOS

ADDITIONAL CODES

300.9	Unspecified Mental Disorder (nonpsychotic)
V71.09	No Diagnosis or Condition on Axis I

PROBLEMS RELATED TO ABUSE OR NEGLECT

V61.21	Physical Abuse of Child (*code 995.5 if focus of attention is on victim*)
V61.21	Sexual Abuse of Child (*code 995.5 if focus of attention is on victim*)
V61.21	Neglect of Child (*code 995.5 if focus of attention is on victim*)
V61.1	Physical Abuse of Adult (*code 995.81 if focus of attention is on victim*)
V61.1	Sexual Abuse of Adult (*code 995.81 if focus of attention is on victim*)

ADDITIONAL CONDITIONS THAT MAY BE A FOCUS OF CLINICAL ATTENTION

V15.81	Noncompliance With Treatment
V65.2	Malingering
V71.01	Adult Antisocial Behavior
V71.02	Child or Adolescent Antisocial Behavior
V62.89	Borderline Intellectual Functioning
	Note: This is coded on Axis II.
780.9	Age-Related Cognitive Decline
V62.82	Bereavement
V62.3	Academic Problem
V62.2	Occupational Problem
313.82	Identity Problem
V62.89	Religious or Spiritual Problem
V62.4	Acculturation Problem
V62.89	Phase of Life Problem

799.9	Diagnosis or Condition Deferred on Axis I
V71.09	No Diagnosis on Axis II
799.9	Diagnosis Deferred on Axis II

MULTIAXIAL SYSTEM

Axis I	Clinical Disorders Other Conditions That May Be a Focus of Clinical Attention	Axis III	General Medical Conditions
Axis II	Personality Disorders Mental Retardation	Axis IV	Psychosocial and Environmental Problems
		Axis V	Global Assessment of Functioning

Subject Index

Note: Page numbers followed by f indicate figures; those followed by t indicate tables. Specific drugs are listed under the generic name in the Drug Index.

Drug Index

Note: Page numbers in **boldface** indicate main discussions. General categories of drugs and drug families (e.g., Antidepressants; Benzodiazepines) are listed in the subject index.